Contents

About the Authors

Basant Pradhan, M.D. works in the Cooper University Health Care, Camden, New Jersey, in the Departments of Psychiatry and Pediatrics where he also serves as the interim chief of Psychiatry and the founding medical director of the neuro-modulation interventions and disorder-specific Yoga and Mindfulness Based Cognitive Therapy (Y-MBCT) programs. In his premedical career, he was a yogi/monk in a monastery in India. In addition to extensive training in psychiatry and psychotherapies, he has trained in clinical neurology, clinical psychology, and cognitive neurosciences which greatly inspire him to combine psychotherapy with brain science and spirituality for diagnostic and treatment purposes. His clinical and research work since 2001 has focused on the development and application of the standardized Yoga and meditation modules as stand-alone treatments and also in combination with medications and neuro-modulation interventions (TMS, Ketamine, ECT) for many chronic and often difficult-to-treat neuropsychiatric conditions, such as treatment-resistant depression, PTSD, psychosis, addictive disorders, and also cognitive disorders such as dyslexia and Huntington's disease. His research has advanced the understanding about neurobiology and therapeutics of the neuropsychiatric disorders and also is aimed at clarifying the pros and cons of psychiatric medications for the young. He has been awarded with the *Institutional Bronze Medal* from the prime minister of India and has been listed in the registry of the *Marquis: Who's Who in America.* His research has received grant awards from organizations like the National Institute on Aging (NIA/NIH), the Brain & Behavior Research Foundation (NARSAD), and the Huntington Study Group, USA. He has lectured at national and international events and published his research widely. Also, he has served the executive council of many reputed organizations, such as the *Group for the Advancement of Psychiatry* (GAP) and the *National Caucus on Integrative Psychiatry*.

Narsimha R. Pinninti, M.D. is a professor of Psychiatry at Rowan University School of Osteopathic Medicine and also medical director of CCBHC, Oaks Integrated Care, both in New Jersey. He oversees the CCBHC and is working to create a system of care for integrating and coordinating care for individuals with serious mental illnesses and substance abuse issues. As part of this effort, he works with Dr. Pradhan and Dr. Rathod to bring improvements in system of care and adapt new psychosocial treatments, such as cognitive behavioral therapy for psychosis and Yoga and Mindfulness Based Cognitive therapy (Y-MBCT) and TIMBER in real-world situations. In addition, his efforts also include training staff in various evidence-based treatments and mindfulness-based meditative practices to reduce stress, to improve health, and to engage with the clients. As a psychiatrist, he runs an ambulatory detox unit and also provides psychiatric services in day hospitalization programs and outpatient program. He is the course director for CBT training for psychiatric residents; has authored a number of papers in peer-reviewed journals, book chapters, and books; and has been an invited speaker nationally.

Shanaya Rathod, M.D. is a professor, consultant psychiatrist, and director of Research at the Southern Health NHS Foundation Trust, UK. She is a visiting professor to the University of Portsmouth and the mental health clinical lead for Wessex Academic Health Science Network and Wessex Clinical Research Network. She is also the trustee to the Centre for Applied Research and Evaluation International Foundation. Following her postgraduate medical education, she has completed a doctorate in medicine and certificate course in Managing Health Services with the Institute of Healthcare Management and acquired a certificate of advance medical leader with the British Association of Medical Managers and masters in Leadership. She has been a fellow with the National Institute for Health and Care Excellence. She has influenced national strategy through her leadership and research over the years and has held a number of leadership roles in the NHS in medical and clinical management. She has a particular interest in developing effective care pathways in mental health services to improve patient outcomes and experience and the cultural and religious aspects of psychopathology of mental illness. She has received grants to explore and improve these areas further. She has published books, book chapters, and papers in peer-reviewed journals and lectured extensively at national and international events. She is a recipient of national and international awards.

Part I

Trauma and the Traumatic Memories (TMs): Manifestations, Mechanisms and Implications

Traumatic Memories and the Spectrum of Their Expressions

1

1.1 Introduction

Trauma and adversities are ubiquitous in society, the awareness and recognition of which has improved significantly in today's culture. The current millennium is about globalization, information explosion, and social media. Global conflict, natural disasters, poverty, and ongoing abuse of human rights have resulted in more numbers of individuals being exposed to trauma. The popular social media, networks, and the 24-hour news broadcasts play a major role in amplifying the impact of traumatic events in the world by exposing its audience instantly to the traumas that are occurring all over the world. In the era of newsprint, people had control over what and when they consumed the news. The digital media and ubiquitous use of cell phones are feeding constant barrage of news, which may be negative, over which the individual has limited control.

There is a growing awareness and recognition of the impact of trauma on the physical and psychological well-being of individuals and communities. In addition to direct trauma exposure, there is secondary (vicarious) trauma of working with the individuals exposed to the trauma, as in the field of mental health, the first responders to trauma events [1] or interpreters working in a therapeutic setting with asylum seekers and refugees [2]. Direct or vicarious exposure to trauma imposes enormous physical, emotional, social, and financial burden on the individuals, the communities, and also the health system. Compared to other professionals, mental healthcare providers are exposed to trauma (both direct and vicarious) on a more consistent basis, and given the deeper relational nature of their work with these clients, they are much more severely affected. Despite this high exposure to trauma and risk of vicarious trauma, more so in the mental healthcare professionals, ironically adequate attention is not being paid to build resilience in them [3].

There are some reports of positive changes in therapists and staff working with traumatized individuals, and these need to be studied and understood better [4].

B. Pradhan et al., *TIMBER Psychotherapy*,
https://doi.org/10.1007/978-3-030-20648-2_1

1.2 The Many Facets of Trauma and the Spectrum of Their Expression

Trauma is a rather complex topic with many facets to it. When it comes to trauma, no two individuals are exactly alike with their symptoms. The clinical example of two siblings described below illustrates how two individuals suffering from the same trauma can have two quite different trauma trajectories. Two female siblings, born a year and half apart, had similar childhood traumatic experiences in form of parental neglect, verbal, physical, as well as sexual abuse coupled with a lack of positive role model in their life. The older sibling went on to develop complex PTSD and bipolar disorder, while the younger one developed generalized anxiety disorder, panic disorder, and polysubstance dependence on alcohol, opioids, and the likes. Despite the fact that the two siblings were only a year and half apart and were raised in the same household where they underwent abuse and neglect, their symptoms and life trajectories turned out to be very different. For example, the older sibling went on to complete college education, had a career as a nurse, entered into a relationship, and had a child. However, her symptoms began interfering in her life significantly when she began to raise this child: her parental role triggered traumatic memories with accompanying distress and dysfunctions. On the other hand, the younger sibling's difficulties began in her high school due to drug use: she dropped out, entered a life of homelessness, polysubstance dependence, became sexually exploited by men and even became incarcerated for drug-related crimes, and was mandated to receive treatment for her multiple health conditions.

An understanding of these complexities of trauma, its various sequelae, and the mechanisms that lead to these helps us to tailor the therapeutic interventions to the psychiatric conditions at hand. This is an evolving field, and for the purpose of our discussion, trauma can be viewed from four different aspects with respect to the nature of trauma and the type of exposure:

1. Single traumatic episode versus repetitive trauma
2. Exposure trauma at the level of individual or at a mass level such as mass shootings
3. Trauma in interpersonal settings and perpetuated by someone with whom the victim has an established relationship
4. Impersonal trauma such as natural disasters

In addition to the individual vulnerability and protective factors, the developmental age at which trauma occurs and the support systems that are available to mitigate the impact of trauma largely determine the trajectories and outcomes for the individuals afflicted with trauma. The fact that majority of individuals exposed to trauma are able deal with it without psychiatric sequela attests to the inherent resilience of the human brain. The sequelae to trauma can be varied and should be viewed on a spectrum. At one end of this spectrum are the individuals who do not have symptoms; on the contrary, the trauma is a growth experience for them, and

TIMBER Psychotherapy

Basant Pradhan • Narsimha R. Pinninti
Shanaya Rathod

TIMBER Psychotherapy

For PTSD, Depression and Traumatic Psychosis

Springer

Basant Pradhan
Department of Psychiatry
Cooper University Hospital
Camden, NJ
USA

Narsimha R. Pinninti
Department of Psychiatry
Rowan University SOM Department of Psychiatry
Cherry Hill, NJ
USA

Shanaya Rathod
Antelope House
Southern Health NHS Foundation Trust
Southampton
UK

ISBN 978-3-030-20647-5 ISBN 978-3-030-20648-2 (eBook)
https://doi.org/10.1007/978-3-030-20648-2

This Springer imprint is published by the registered company Springer Nature Switzerland AG
The registered company address is: Gewerbestrasse 11, 6330 Cham, Switzerland

3/16/2019: "This manual is a scientific treatise on the powerful impact of a meditation-based psychotherapy on the difficult-to-treat conditions such as chronic PTSD, resistant depression, and traumatic psychosis. Firmly anchored in the contemporary cognitive neurosciences, fusing the Eastern mysticism with the pragmatism of cognitive behavioral therapy, this compelling textbook urges for a paradigm shift in trauma therapy. Truly, it opens up new vistas of thought and praxis for the afflicted as well as for the healers at all levels of experience. I am sure this will also add a lot of value to the current literature on this topic."

—Afzal Javed, M.D., President Elect, *World Psychiatric Association*

3/20/2019: "Trauma has increasingly been identified as a key issue contributing to mental health problems ranging beyond PTSD to depression, substance misuse, and psychosis. Complex PTSD is now a term used in ICD-11 to describe conditions arising from repetitive trauma and is much more descriptive than terms, such as personality disorder, previously used. This book is therefore very timely in describing new approaches which have been subjected to scientific evaluation that address these effects of trauma."

—David Kingdon, M.D., *Professor of Psychiatry, University of South Hampton, UK*

3/23/2019: "It has been my privilege to witness and follow Dr. Pradhan's groundbreaking work for some time. This collaboration with Drs. Pinninti and Rathod is his latest contribution and evolution of the Yoga and Mindfulness Based Cognitive Therapy (Y-MBCT) models for which TIMBER is the prototype. This book presents the compelling rationale for these innovative models, as well as their underpinning in cognitive psychology, spirituality, and neuroscience. The emphasis on cultural context is particularly important, given the cultural origins of the model and its sensitivity to cultural adaptation in its programmatic implementation."

—Andres J. Pumariega, M.D., Professor and Chief, *Division of Child and Adolescent Psychiatry, University of Florida College of Medicine*

Dedicated to all our clients....

... for trusting us with their deepest thoughts and feelings
... for sharing their journey on the TIMBER path with us,
... for practicing meditation with us during their therapy sessions,
... for their resilience and mindfulness that kept us inspired and mindful throughout our work with them in the clinics and in this book project

We feel privileged and honored to be part of their journey of recovery...

Foreword

Trauma is a universal experience. All of us go through experiencing trauma one way or the other through our lifetime, but the type of trauma and our responses are modified according to a number of factors. Neither all people will respond in the same way to trauma nor will they respond to the same treatment in the same way. Over the past few decades, there has been a plethora of therapies in dealing with and managing trauma-based experiences. As societies have changed social capital and social support, systems have changed too which has created additional problems in accessing therapies which are culturally appropriate and suitable. There are a number of psychiatric conditions which can be caused by traumatic experiences and also contribute to persistence of traumatic memories. There is no doubt that some memories can become pathological and affect psychopathology and individual responses. The symptoms too get affected by the experiences and idioms of distress. These traumatic memories and experiences can perpetuate pathology and suffering.

In this volume, Pradhan and colleagues describe therapies which target these memories.

Unlike cognitive behavioral therapy, TIMBER (*Trauma Interventions using Mindfulness Based Extinction and Reconsolidation* of memories) psychotherapy described in this volume offers a novel, evidence-based, and biomarker (D-serine)-informed mindfulness-based CBT approach. This tackles some of the existing treatment gaps. Combining the new therapy, mindfulness-based tools with cognitive behavioral therapy, provides a unique way to manage traumatic memories and experiences. TIMBER includes various modified CBT interventions, such as mindfulness-based graded exposure therapy (MB-GET) and cognitive reprocessing, and these can be used as therapist-based and self-help approaches so that trauma memories and their expressions in clients' daily life can be managed. Reducing stress, managing distress, and improving coping in the clients, their carers, and others are important steps forward. After having established its efficacy in chronic PTSD and depression, extending this approach's application to other psychiatric conditions, such as traumatic psychosis, drug addiction, and borderline personality disorder, may well prove to be successful.

This treatment manual aims to introduce the practitioners and the clients to a stepwise approach. The authors deserve our thanks and congratulations for bringing together these approaches so that our patients get the best approach and best results. I hope that therapist dealing with trauma will find this approach helpful but that all therapists will learn from this approach.

Dinesh Bhugra
Mental health and Cultural Diversity IoPPN,
Kings College
London, UK

Preface

Trauma, Traumatic Memories, and TIMBER

Trauma is probably one of the most devastating sufferings of the human mind that has a wide array of health consequences, both mental and physical. The impact of trauma is now recognized more widely than ever due to globalization, widespread social media, and the inadequacies of our existing systems to protect individuals and communities. Trauma may result in many serious and often chronic mental health conditions, such as post-traumatic stress disorder (PTSD), treatment-resistant depression, traumatic psychosis, drug addiction, borderline personality disorder, etc. Cutting-edge translational research, more so after year 2000, reveals that in these conditions, pathological trauma memories (TMs) become ingrained into distinct brain areas through conditioned learning. These TMs lay at the core of the psychopathologies and influence the formation, maintenance, and expression of the major symptoms in these often chronic disorders. Some aspects of memory, in particular the involuntary expressions of the trauma/fear memories, as seen in PTSD or traumatic psychosis or the likes, can be very problematic and pathogenetic. As Irving [1] elegantly points it out:

> *Your memory is a monster; you forget - it doesn't. It simply files things away. It keeps things for you, or hides things from you - and summons them to your recall with a will of its own. You think you have a memory; but it has you!*

The victims of trauma are truly the captives of their pathologically ingrained trauma memories which dictate their lives.

Unfortunately, TMs have been so far neglected or rather unexplored despite the tremendous influence TMs play in the formation, maintenance, and expression of the major symptoms in these disorders. One explanation for the suboptimal responses to the current treatment options for these conditions is that many of them do not specifically target the TMs. A renewed focus on these aspects can lead to the development of more efficacious and evidence-based interventions and, therefore, has much to offer for the scientists, patients, and therapists alike. Cognitive behavioral therapy (CBT), despite its established efficacy and utility, does not yet have a psychobiological-based platform to address trauma memories comprehensively and so can result in vulnerability to relapse of symptoms, although many clients may improve initially.

TIMBER (*Trauma Interventions* using *Mindfulness Based Extinction* and *Reconsolidation* of memories) psychotherapy is a novel, evidence-based, and biomarker-informed (plasma D-serine, [2]) mindfulness-based CBT approach developed by Basant Pradhan, MD, who attempts to address some of the existing treatment gaps [3, 4]. Technically, TIMBER belongs to the emerging category of *third wave CBT* [5, 6]. In addition to incorporating the mindfulness-based tools, TIMBER involves the use of modified CBT interventions, such as mindfulness-based graded exposure therapy (MB-GET) and cognitive reprocessing, both of which in a self-help and user-friendly format target and attempt to change the trauma memories and their expressions in clients' daily life. The wellness component of TIMBER is aimed at stress reduction and better coping in the clients, in their significant others, as well as in the therapist, while its illness component targets the trauma memories and their expressions. Its experiential aspects and fidelity of its application are enhanced by the therapist practicing with the clients during the therapy sessions, which promotes therapist's empathy and expertise in applying this model as well as reduces stress. The translational concepts and the customized and targeted interventions done in TIMBER have led to a paradigm shift toward a broader and deeper understanding of chronic PTSD, depression, and traumatic psychosis. The efficacy of TIMBER has been studied in placebo-controlled randomized studies for chronic PTSD and depression in adults [2, 7], in a pilot study in adolescents [8], and also in a multicentric case series in traumatic psychosis [9]. After having established the efficacies in chronic PTSD, treatment-resistant depression, and traumatic psychosis, extending TIMBER's application to other conditions, such as drug addiction, borderline personality disorder is likely to enhance the outcomes for individuals afflicted with these conditions. One of the criticisms levelled against psychotherapy today, particularly CBT, is for the process being technical with less emphasis on the experience. The emphasis in this book is primarily on the experiential aspects of TIMBER with theoretical and didactic information included to supplement this experience. In doing so, our goal is to enhance the self-efficacy of the clients and their family members in addition to delivering TIMBER in culturally sensitive manner.

This treatment manual serves for the practitioners and the clients as a step-by-step guide on TIMBER psychotherapy and has been organized into *three parts consisting of seven chapters*. Cogently describing the important connection between the traumatic memories giving rise to PTSD, treatment-resistant depression, and traumatic psychosis and emphasizing upon the complex relationship between each of these conditions perpetuating the trauma further in the course of time as well as in various settings including in the treatment situations, the descriptions, the data, and the illustrations in this clinical manual unfold in the following seven chapters.

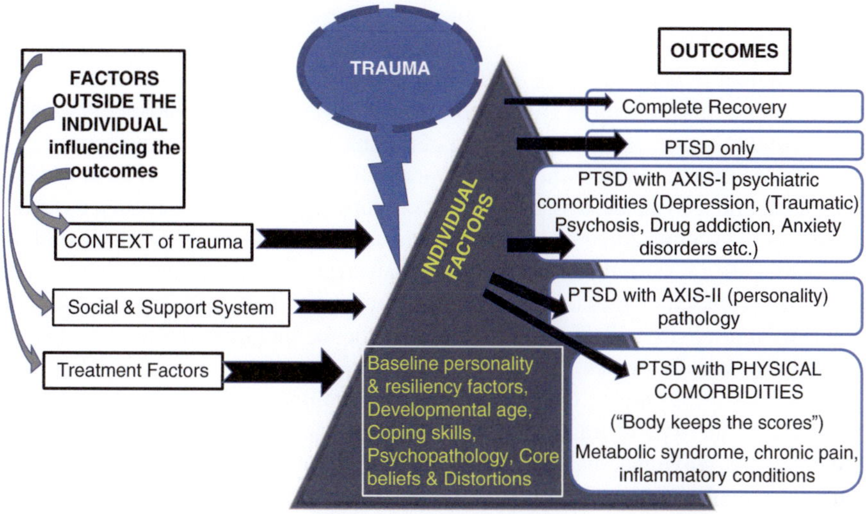

Fig. 1.1 Trauma, its various trajectories, and the factors mediating the clinical outcomes

more often than not, it makes them very empathic trauma counselors [5]. However, at the other end can be the individuals with multitudes of health conditions, both mental and physical, all emanating from the trauma and many of which can have devastating and sometimes lifelong impacts. The many trajectories of trauma, the spectrum of its manifestations, as well as the mediating factors are depicted in Fig. 1.1.

The mental health conditions in this spectrum include the post-traumatic stress disorder (PTSD), other anxiety disorders including the dissociative disorders, major depressive disorder, various substance abuse disorders, psychotic disorders like traumatic psychosis (conceptualized as a subgroup of schizophrenia), attention deficit hyperactivity disorder (ADHD), and borderline personality disorders (BLPD) [6–8]. However, this book focusses on three primary diagnoses: PTSD, psychosis, particularly traumatic psychosis, and major depressive disorder that is often comorbid with PTSD in the trauma settings. As a specific therapy targeting these, TIMBER (*Trauma Interventions* using *Mindfulness-Based Extinction and Reconsolidation* of memories) psychotherapy has evidences on its efficacy in all three conditions [9–13]. In addition, the authors' clinical experiences and unpublished data from ongoing research suggest the effectiveness of TIMBER in a variety of other psychiatric conditions such as addictive disorders, but those are not covered in this book.

Trauma that is perpetrated in childhood such as physical and sexual trauma can be categorized as primary, secondary, and tertiary, based on the traumatic contexts of the individuals—from their natural support system to the broad health systems of care, in particular mental health system. Primary trauma involves the index traumatic event experienced by the individual. Secondary trauma occurs when the primary support system of the individual further traumatizes the individual by invalidation of their trauma. For example, an 8-year-old girl sexually abused by her stepfather confides in her mother who chooses not to believe her and allows the sexual trauma to continue, thus causing secondary trauma. On the other hand, the presence of a trusted adult in childhood who has always been available emotionally to the child mitigates the adverse impact of trauma and increases the resilience [14]. The tertiary trauma occurs where the mental health system further traumatizes the individual either by insensitive assessment or inappropriate responses such as invalidation of the trauma and the sequelae. The results of secondary and tertiary trauma are chronicity of symptoms, functional impairment, and disability. More importantly, it severely damages the ability of the trauma victim to trust any parenting or authority figures, thus making it much harder for the therapists to build a trusting relationship and do the healing-related work.

The pathogenic impact of trauma varies depending on mainly three groups of factors, e.g., the type of trauma, the ensuing responses and the extent of resiliency factors in the individual, and the availability and extent of support systems are present to help deal with the trauma. All these factors are depicted in Fig. 1.1. The pathways from childhood adversity to various sequelae are still being elucidated but include biological and psychological mechanisms. Childhood psychosocial adversity is shown to cause disruption of central neural networks, neuroendocrine stress dysregulation, and chronic inflammation, among other changes, and these lead to adverse outcomes, including physical conditions like diabetes, heart disease, cancers, in addition to psychiatric illnesses [15]. An online study of more than 30,000 adults in the United Kingdom showed that the relation between environmental stressors, including trauma, and mental health symptoms was strongly mediated by a range of psychological processes, such as self-blame, rumination, and absence of coping ([16]).

1.3 Impact of Trauma in Early Life and Risk of PTSD, Depression, and Psychosis

Trauma, especially early life trauma, is a risk factor for the development of PTSD, major depressive disorder, and traumatic psychosis [17]. Researchers at University of Bristol, United Kingdom [18], analyzed data from the *Avon Longitudinal Study of Parents and Children*, a large population-based birth cohort in the United Kingdom of women who had an expected delivery date between April 1, 1991, and December 31, 1992. This large sample comprised of 14,775 live births and the critical findings was that the children and adolescents who are exposed to any kind of trauma before the age of 17 are more likely to have psychotic experiences by age 18. This study also demonstrated a dose-response relationship between the severity of trauma and the likelihood of psychopathology (i.e., psychosis). Exposure to three or more types of trauma by the age of 17 was associated with a 4.7-fold increase in the odds of having psychotic experiences. Additionally, exposure to trauma during early and middle childhood as well as adolescence was associated with a higher risk of developing psychotic experiences than exposure within only one or two of these periods. These researchers opine that "...assuming the association is accurate and causal, a substantial proportion of participants would not have developed psychotic experiences if they had not been exposed to traumatic experiences during childhood."

A number of other studies as well have demonstrated clear associations between childhood trauma exposure and the development of psychotic disorders [17, 19–27], thereby demonstrating that trauma is a factor in the development of not only PTSD but also psychosis. Similarly, Mueser et al. [28] suggest that PTSD may mediate the relationship between trauma and severity of the symptom or impairments in severe mental illnesses. In this model, PTSD and psychotic disorder are seen as distinct disorders that interact with one another creating a compounded risk for increased psychotic and PTSD symptoms. In contrast, in another model proposed by Morrison et al. [29], PTSD and psychosis are seen as similar entities that are part of a broader spectrum of reactions to trauma. Emphasizing upon the adverse impacts of the childhood trauma exposure, Andrianarisoa et al. [30] report that in schizophrenia, quality of life is independently impacted by childhood trauma, depression, and negative symptoms.

The relationship between childhood adversity, trauma, and treatment-resistant depression (TRD) merits a discussion. Lindert et al. [31] in a meta-analysis of 19 studies that included 115,579 subjects reported that childhood physical and sexual abuse are associated with higher incidence of depression (the combined odds ratios were 2.04 for sexual abuse and 1.49 for physical abuse) and anxiety disorders (the combined odds ratios were 2.52 for sexual abuse and 1.70 for physical abuse) in these adults [31]. Further, Kaplan and Klinetob [32] demonstrated that in treatment-resistant depression (TRD), childhood adversity and trauma were associated with poorer clinical course, including earlier age of onset, more persistence of the episodes, and also more recurrences. Their conclusion was that childhood adversity was common among patients with TRD and was associated with poor clinical course, psychosis, and suicide attempts as well.

1.4 Shared Psychopathologies in PTSD, Traumatic Psychosis, and Treatment-Resistant Depression

There are many similarities of PTSD and psychotic disorders like schizophrenia. In fact, the symptoms of PTSD and psychosis can exist together as part of a spectrum of experiences related to traumatic events [29, 33]. As mentioned before, although opinions differ about the exact relationship between trauma, PTSD, and psychosis, consensus does exist that trauma can induce symptoms of psychosis and vice versa. For example, in people with psychosis, the experience of hospitalization can produce emotional, cognitive, and behavioral responses that may meet diagnostic criteria for PTSD [34, 35]. These evidences indicate a shared psychopathology.

Many people with PTSD, especially those with complex trauma (defined as exposure to multiple and severe traumatic events during childhood which are often of an invasive and interpersonal nature, more details in Chap. 5), can present with secondary psychotic features [36, 37] in the form of hallucinations and delusions in addition to the usual symptoms of PTSD. These hallucinations, with respect to their contents, are generally related to the theme of the traumatic events but can be accompanied by non-trauma-related contents as well. The delusions have typically persecutory and/or paranoid contents [38]. In PTSD, the intensities of paranoid thinking and agitation are much higher in people who experience these psychotic features compared to who don't, and most clinicians lack therapeutic success with this complex clinical condition [27]. Although the etiological relationships between trauma and PTSD are clear, the pathway from trauma to psychosis and depression needs more clarity. Similarly, the various factors contributing to this trauma-PTSD-depression-psychosis diathesis are yet to be evaluated in rigorous research studies and need to be understood more comprehensively.

The relationship between trauma and psychosis has been both causal and intricate. Zubin and Spring [39] in their *stress-vulnerability model* of schizophrenia have tried to explain this, at least in part. They emphasized that the common denominator across all the perspectives trying to explain psychosis (in particular, schizophrenia) was that of a vulnerability such as bad genes, problematic internal environment, abnormal neurophysiology emanating from the traumatic experiences, the presence of specific diseases or perinatal complications, stressful family experiences and other life events, etc. Interestingly, this model sees these vulnerabilities as *permanent, unchangeable states*, whereas symptoms in schizophrenia are seen in this model as episodic and presenting in response to certain "challengers to adaptation." Certain situations may provoke a temporary crisis in coping which may result in an episode of schizophrenia. A person's ability to cope with such events is shaped by their vulnerabilities, learning, and resilience factors. Illness models like these help to reduce stigma and aim to promote psychological and environmental interventions to support coping; they also emphasize the need for preventative measures once the vulnerabilities are identified.

Based on the explanations of Zubin and Spring, Kingdon and Turkington have suggested four subgroups of psychosis: (1) traumatic, (2) drug-related, (3) anxiety-related, and (4) sensitivity psychosis. These subgroups arose from clinical observation and surveys of different populations and actually are formulations informed and derived from a CBT (cognitive-behavioral therapy) based understanding of psychosis. They are based on a bio-psychosocial as well as stress-vulnerability model of people's experiences [40, 41]. These subgroups may overcome some of the difficulties experienced in other classifications as they describe factors influencing onset of psychosis and can be expected to be stable over the course of episodes or where enduring.

Traumatic memories (TMs) remain the common feature in PTSD, traumatic psychosis, and major depressive disorder, particularly treatment-resistant type [6, 32]. In these conditions, pathologically ingrained trauma memories (TMs) lay at the core of the psychopathologies which become ingrained into distinct brain areas through conditioned learning mediated by the hippocampus, amygdala, prefrontal cortex, and basal ganglia along with the brain stem and hypothalamus-pituitary axis [10, 11]. More details on the TMs can be found in Chap. 2. Ironically, the existing etiological models of PTSD, traumatic psychosis, and major depressive disorder do not consider TMs as critical in maintaining pathology in these conditions. Like some other researchers [42], we are of the opinion that in these disorders, TMs play a critical role in the formation, maintenance, and expression of the major symptoms, e.g., intrusive thoughts, flashbacks, hallucinations, avoidance, numbing, dissociation, hyperarousal, and affect dysregulation. As trauma memories lay at the core in etiopathogenesis of conditions like post-traumatic stress disorder (PTSD), TRD, and traumatic psychosis, using pharmacological and cognitive-behavioral treatments that specifically target trauma memories can improve the outcome.

1.5 Therapeutic Role of Meditation in PTSD and Traumatic Psychosis

Therapeutic role of meditation in psychiatric conditions that include PTSD, depression, and psychosis has been shown in many studies [43, 44]. In another recent randomized controlled trial [45] involving 203 veterans with a current diagnosis of PTSD resulting from traumatic event(s) experienced during active military service, researchers compared the efficacy of transcendental meditation with that of exposure therapy as well as that of health education. In this head-to-head comparison, these researchers found that both transcendental meditation and exposure therapy (each comprising of 12 sessions over 12 weeks) were superior to health education at reducing clinician- and patient-rated PTSD symptoms, as well as depressive symptoms; 61% of veterans receiving transcendental meditation, 42% of those receiving exposure therapy, and 32% of those receiving health education showed a clinically relevant improvement in symptoms (defined as at least a 10-point drop in their Clinician-Administered PTSD Scale (CAPS) scores). In this study, the meditation and health education sessions were provided in group settings, while the exposure therapy was given in one-on-one settings. These researchers concluded that meditation training could have a substantial effect on health as an adjunct to the standard of care and might have considerable value in improving the quality of life for military service members who have been victims of trauma.

1.6 TIMBER Psychotherapy for Trauma Memories

TIMBER (*Trauma Interventions* using *Mindfulness-Based Extinction and Reconsolidation* of memories), as the name suggests, is a trauma-specific mindfulness-based cognitive-behavioral therapy (CBT) which was developed by Basant Pradhan. Technically, TIMBER belongs to the emerging category of *third wave CBT* [46]. In addition to incorporating the mindfulness-based tools, TIMBER involves the use of modified CBT interventions, such as mindfulness-based graded exposure therapy (MB-GET) and cognitive reprocessing, both of which in a self-help and user-friendly format target and attempt to change the trauma memories and their expressions in clients' daily life. In its initial application, TIMBER was found efficacious in chronic and treatment refractory PTSD in the youth [9] and adults [12]. Subsequently its indication was extended to traumatic psychosis [10] and chronic depression [13] as well. TIMBER is based on a more recent neurobiological understanding of trauma memories and uses a balanced combination of trauma memory extinction (i.e., gradual diminishing of a conditioned response over time as a person learns to uncouple a response from a stimulus) and trauma memory reconsolidation (i.e., retrieval of memories to strengthen, add, or remove information, and then update them) approaches. These are two fundamental learning methods that play a crucial role in maintenance of trauma memories, which are increasingly being recognized as the core pathologies in PTSD and traumatic psychosis. The Chap. 2 deals with the role of trauma memories in extensive detail. The unique and standardized methodology of TIMBER keeps the trauma memory retrieval controlled and the hyperarousal symptoms not too overwhelming so that it does not cause overflooding and re-traumatization for clients that is seen more often than not in some other exposure-based treatment approaches. TIMBER does so by incorporating a broad array of interventions that include Yoga, mindfulness, and mindfulness-based graded exposure therapy (MB-GET, [11]) which is a type of modified CBT. Another key aspect of TIMBER is that it first ensures skill building in the client and caregivers by formal training in Yoga and meditation by the use of the StaMP (Standardized Meditation Program) protocol which forms its *wellness component*. After these skills are achieved, it specifically focuses on changing the expressions of trauma memories in the client's daily life which constitute its *illness- or disorder-specific component*.

TIMBER has been used both as a stand-alone therapy as well as in combination with psychotropic medications, both oral and parenteral such as ketamine infusion. TIMBER psychotherapy augmented with a single dose of ketamine infusion at a subanesthetic dose (0.5 mg/kg) has produced 80–85% response in two randomized controlled trials with 2-year longitudinal follow-up design [12, 13]. In another small study [10], eight sessions (30–45 min duration each) of *TIMBER* were administered over a period of 14 weeks to five female clients with non-affective psychosis. Out of these five clients, one was adolescent, three were middle aged adults, and one was elderly. Among these five clients, two (one adolescent and one adult) achieved remission of psychotic symptoms, and two adults had significant reduction in their symptoms. Although preliminary, these data show that *TIMBER* can be a feasible therapeutic option and can be effective in inducing remission of psychotic symptoms. Detailed evidence for biomarkers (plasma D-Serine) for TIMBER will be further detailed later in the book.

1.7 Conclusion and Future Directions

Deeply ingrained traumatic memories (TMs) lay at the core of the psychopathologies in PTSD, traumatic psychosis, and treatment-resistant depression (TRD), especially in the settings of trauma. Considering the huge public health burden of these conditions, their frequent chronicity, comorbidity, as well treatment refractoriness, there is a dire need to develop effective, evidence-based, integrated, and multidisciplinary care models for these conditions. Research suggesting significantly better outcomes in PTSD, depression, or psychosis when treated early in the course of these illnesses has led to efforts to provide coordinated, multispecialty care as soon as possible to individuals who experience a traumatic event or those who develop an episode of psychosis for the first time. Novel interventions like TIMBER that aim to address how trauma affects the mechanisms underlying the development of PTSD, treatment-resistant depression, as well as the psychotic experiences could improve mental health outcomes in these often chronic and difficult to treat conditions, and replicating these in multiple clinical settings will remain a priority in our future work related to this.

References

1. Flannery RB Jr. Treating psychological trauma in first responders: a multi-modal paradigm. Psychiatry Q. 2015;86(2):261–7.
2. Splevins KA, Cohen K, Joseph S, Murray C, Bowley J. Vicarious posttraumatic growth among interpreters. Qual Health Res. 2010;20(12):1705–16.
3. Sweeney A, Fison B, Kennedy A, et al. A paradigm shift: relationships in trauma-informed mental health services. B J Psych Adv. 2018;24(5):319–33.
4. Linley PA, et al. Trauma work, sense of coherence, and positive and negative changes in therapists. Psychother Psychosom. 2005;74(3):185–8.
5. Khanna S, Greyson B. Near-death experiences and posttraumatic growth. J Nerv Ment Dis. 2015;203(10):749–55.
6. Mandelli P, Serretti, et al. The role of specific early trauma in adult depression: a meta-analysis of published literature. Childhood trauma and adult depression. Eur Psychiatry. 2015;30(6):665–80.
7. Koyuncu A, Çelebi F, Ertekin E. Attention deficit and hyperactivity in social anxiety disorder: relationship with trauma history and impulsivity. ADHD: Attention Deficit and Hyperactivity Disorders. 2016;8(2):95–100.
8. Golier JA, Yehuda R, Bierer LM, Mitropoulou V, New AS, Schmeidler J, et al. The relationship of borderline personality disorder to posttraumatic stress disorder and traumatic events. Am J Psychiatry. 2003;160:2018–24.
9. Pradhan BK, Gray RM, Parikh T, Akkireddi P, Pumariega A. Trauma Interventions using Mindfulness Based Extinction and Reconsolidation (TIMBER) as monotherapy for chronic PTSD in adolescents: a pilot study. Adolescent Psychiat. 2015;5(2):125–31.
10. Pradhan BK, Pinninti NR, Rathod S, editors. Brief interventions for psychosis: a clinical compendium. Switzerland: Springer; 2016.
11. Pradhan BK. Clinical considerations for youth with trauma & TIMBER psychotherapy as an emerging evidence-based treatment. In: Blanco RF, Bogacki DF, editors. Prescriptions for children with learning and adjustment problems: a consultant's desk reference. Springfield, Illinois: Charles C. Thomas; 2017.
12. Pradhan BK, Wainer IW, Moaddel R, Torjman MC, Goldberg M, Sabia M, Parikh T, Pumariega AJ. Trauma interventions using mindfulness based extinction and reconsolidation (TIMBER) psychotherapy prolong the therapeutic effects of single ketamine infusion on post-traumatic stress disorder and comorbid depression: a pilot randomized, placebo-controlled, cross-over clinical trial. Asia Pac J Clin Trials Nerv Syst Dis. 2017;2(3):80–90.
13. Pradhan BK, Mitrev L, Moaddel R, Wainer I. D-serine is a biomarker for clinical response in (R, S)-ketamine treatment of post-traumatic stress disorder and co-morbid depression. Biochim Biophys Acta. 2018;S1570-9639(18):30035–9.

14. Bellis MA, et al. Does continuous trusted adult support in childhood impart life-course resilience against adverse childhood experiences - a retrospective study on adult health-harming behaviours and mental Well-being. BMC Psychiatry. 2017;17(1):110.
15. Berens AE, et al. Biological embedding of childhood adversity: from physiological mechanisms to clinical implications. BMC Med. 2017;15(1):135.
16. Kinderman P, Schwannauer M, Pontin E, Tai S. Psychological processes mediate the impact of familial risk, social circumstances and life events on mental health. PLoS One. 2013;8:e76564.
17. Powers A, Fani N, Cross D, Ressler KJ, Bradley B. Childhood trauma, PTSD, and psychosis: findings from a highly traumatized, minority sample. Child Abuse Negl. 2016;58:111–8. https://doi.org/10.1016/j.chiabu.2016.06.015.
18. Croft J, Heron J, Teufel C, et al. Association of trauma type, age of exposure, and frequency in childhood and adolescence with psychotic experiences in early adulthood. JAMA Psychiat. 2018; https://doi.org/10.1001/jamapsychiatry.2018.3155.
19. Arseneault L, Cannon M, Fisher HL, Polanczyk G, Moffitt TE, Caspi A. Childhood trauma and children's emerging psychotic symptoms: a genetically sensitive longitudinal cohort study. Am J Psychiatry. 2011;168(1):65–72.
20. Bendall S, Jackson HJ, Hulbert CA, McGorry PD. Childhood trauma and psychotic disorders: a systematic, critical review of the evidence. Schizophr Bull. 2008;34(3):568–79.
21. Gaudiano BA, Zimmerman M. Evaluation of evidence for the psychotic subtyping of post-traumatic stress disorder. Br J Psychiatry. 2010a;197(4):326–7.
22. Gaudiano BA, Zimmerman M. The relationship between childhood trauma history and the psychotic subtype of major depression. Acta Psychiatr Scand. 2010b;121(6):462–70. https://doi.org/10.1111/j.1600-0447.2009.01477.x. Epub 2009 Sep 18
23. Morgan C, Fisher H. Environment and schizophrenia: environmental factors in schizophrenia: childhood trauma--a critical review. Schizophr Bull. 2007;33(1):3–10.
24. Read J, van Os J, Morrison AP, Ross CA. Childhood trauma, psychosis and schizophrenia: a literature review with theoretical and clinical implications. Acta Psychiatr Scand. 2005;112(5):330–50.
25. Schafer I, Fisher HL. Childhood trauma and posttraumatic stress disorder in patients with psychosis: clinical challenges and emerging treatments. Curr Opin Psychiatry. 2011a;24(6):514–8.
26. Schafer I, Fisher HL. Childhood trauma and psychosis - what is the evidence? Dialogues Clin Neurosci. 2011b;13(3):360–5.
27. Varese F, Smeets F, Drukker M, Lieverse R, Lataster T, Viechtbauer W, Read J, van Os J, Bentall RP. Childhood adversities increase the risk of psychosis: a meta-analysis of patient-control, prospective- and cross-sectional cohort studies. Schizophr Bull. 2012;38(4):661–71.
28. Mueser KT, Rosenberg SD, Goodman LA, Trumbetta SL. Trauma, PTSD and the course of schizophrenia: AN interactive model. Schizophr Res. 2002;53:123–43.
29. Morrison A, Frame L, Larkin W. Relationship between trauma and psychosis: a review and integration. Br J Clin Psychol. 2003;42(4):331–53.
30. Andrianarisoa M, Boyer L, Gordin O, et al. Childhood trauma, depression and negative symptoms are independently associated with impaired quality of life in schizophrenia. Results from the national FACE-SZ cohort. Schizophr Res. 2017;185:173–81.
31. Lindert J, von Ehrenstein OS, Grashow R, et al. Sexual and physical abuse in childhood is associated with depression and anxiety over the life course: systematic review and meta-analysis. Int J Public Health. 2014;59(2):359–72.
32. Kaplan MJ, Klinetob NA. Childhood emotional trauma and chronic posttraumatic stress disorder in adult outpatients with treatment-resistant depression. J Nerv Ment Dis. 2000;188(9):596–601.
33. Fleming M, Richards D. The relationship between traumatic reactions and psychosis. Ment Health Pract. 2006;9(9):18–22.
34. Frame L, Morrison A. Causes of PTSD in psychosis. Arch Gen Psychiatry. 2001;58(3):305–6.
35. McGorry P, Chanen A, McCarthy E, et al. Post-traumatic stress disorder following recent onset psychosis: an unrecognized post-psychotic syndrome. J Nerv Ment Dis. 1991;179(5):253–8.

36. Braakman M, Kortmann F, van der Brink W. Validity of post-traumatic stress disorder with secondary features: a review of the evidence. Acta Psychiatr Scand. 2009;119(1):15–24.
37. Katsounari I. Post-traumatic stress disorder and psychosis. Ment Health Pract. 2011;15(4):14–8.
38. Hamner M, Frueh C, Ulmner HG, et al. Psychotic features in chronic posttraumatic stress disorder and schizophrenia. J Nerv Ment Dis. 2000;188(4):217–21.
39. Zubin J, Spring B. Vulnerability: a new view on schizophrenia. J Abnorm Psychol. 1997;86(2):103–26.
40. Kingdon D, Vincent S, Vincent S, Kinoshita Y, Turkington D. Destigmatizing schizophrenia: does changing terminology reduce negative attitudes? Psychiatr Bull. 2008;32(12):419–22.
41. Rathod S, Irfan M, Bhargava R, et al. Multinational comparative cross-sectional survey of views of medical students about acceptable terminology and subgroups in schizophrenia. BMJ Open. 2018;8:e021461. https://doi.org/10.1136/bmjopen-2017-021461.
42. Visser RM, Lau-Zhu A, Henson RN, Holmes EA. Multiple memory systems, multiple time points: how science can inform treatment to control the expression of unwanted emotional memories. Phil Trans R Soc B. 2018;373:20170209. https://doi.org/10.1098/rstb.2017.0209
43. Balasubramaniam M, Telles S, Doraiswamy PM. Yoga on our minds: a systematic review of yoga for neuropsychiatric disorders. Front Psych. 2013;3:117. https://doi.org/10.3389/fpsyt.2012.00117.
44. Brown RP, Gerbarg PL. Sudarshan Kriya yogic (SKY) breathing in the treatment of stress, anxiety, and depression: clinical applications and guidelines. J Altern Complement Med. 2005;11(4):711–7.
45. Nidich S, Mills PJ, Rainforth M, et al. Non-trauma-focused meditation versus exposure therapy in veterans with post-traumatic stress disorder: a randomized controlled trial. Lancet Psychiatry. 2018;5(12):p975–86. https://doi.org/10.1016/S2215-0366(18)30384-5.
46. Kahl KG, Winter L, Schweiger U. The third wave of cognitive behavioural therapies. Curr Opin Psychiatry. 2012;25(6):522–8.

Traumatic Memories (TMs): Neurobiology and Implications

2

2.1 Introduction

Memories that have strong emotions (such as fear) associated with them are particularly resistant to decay or forgetting. Some aspects of the memory, in particular, the involuntary expressions of the trauma/fear memories, as seen in PTSD or traumatic psychosis or the likes, can be very problematic and pathogenetic. As Irving [1] elegantly points it out: "Your memory is a monster; you forget—it doesn't. It simply files things away. It keeps things for you, or hides things from you—and summons them to your recall with a will of its own. You think you have a memory; but it has you!"

As briefly mentioned in Chap. 1, more recent evidence suggests that deeply ingrained trauma memories (TMs) lay at the core of the psychopathology and influence the formation, expression and maintenance of key symptoms, such as intrusive thoughts, flashbacks, avoidance, numbing, and hyperarousal. These TMs become systematically ingrained into the brain through conditioned learning mediated by the various brain structures such as hippocampus, amygdala, prefrontal cortex, and basal ganglia along with the brain stem and hypothalamus-pituitary axis [2–4]. The disturbed functionality of the neural circuits involved in the processing and expression of the trauma memories perpetuates these symptoms and is linked not only to the effects of the contexts in which the trauma had originally occurred but also to their subsequent reenactments in the victim's life as well as the individual, social, environmental, and genetic risk factors, which converge on these neural networks. Similarly, we have already discussed the association between trauma, psychosis, and treatment resistant depression (TRD). The existing psychopharmacological and psychotherapeutic treatments are less than optimal with respect to their efficacy [5, 6], and therefore, new models of treatment that incorporate the recent neurobiological research into trauma are needed. New translational research strategies are needed to delineate as well as mechanistically tap into the various trajectories involved in the expression of traumatic memories so that more efficacious and evidence-based interventions can be developed and tested reliably in these often difficult-to-treat conditions.

B. Pradhan et al., *TIMBER Psychotherapy*,
https://doi.org/10.1007/978-3-030-20648-2_2

2.2 Processes Involved in Trauma/Fear Memories

Memory is the neural representation of information. Cognitive neuroscientists define our experiences as *internal representations* of things in our brain and mind. Memory, our ability to remember things/experiences, is the *retention*, *reactivation*, and *reconstruction* of these internal representations and thus plays a crucial role in reproducing our experiences. This information is first registered and acquired (*memory acquisition*) in the internal system and, if strengthened (*memory consolidation*), is eventually stored in a relatively stable manner in our long-term memory. *Memory consolidation* is a process that the brain carries out to convert short-term memories to long-term memories in which the medial temporal lobe plays a key role [7]. Memory consolidation involves the process of neural changes that occur after learning to create the *memory trace* (i.e., the physical change in the nervous system) of an experience. The three stages involved in the formation memory are [8, 9]:

- Registration and encoding
- Storage
- Retrieval

Encoding is defined as the initial registration of the stimuli and their association with other parameters of the experience to perceive and learn the information; storage refers to maintaining the information over time; retrieval is the ability to access information when one needs it. Long-term memory (LTM) operates within the hippocampus with connections to the cortex, thalamus, and other sites in the limbic system. The hippocampus serves an index pointing function to other cortical memory sites where memories are consolidated. The hippocampus is essential for the consolidation of information from short-term to long-term memory, and without the hippocampus, new memories cannot be stored into the LTM, although the hippocampus itself does not seem to store information itself. Although structures in the medial temporal lobe (MTL) appear to be necessary for the establishment of LTM, they may also be involved in further consolidation of information through *higher-order memory*. Consolidation of new memories depends on a crucial phase of protein synthesis and presumably involves two processes at the molecular level: *synaptic consolidation* and *system consolidation*. The former involves a process of protein synthesis in the medial temporal lobe (MTL), whereas the latter transforms the MTL-dependent memory into an MTL-independent memory over the duration of months to years [10]. In recent years, the new studies on memory reconsolidation have led to re-evaluate the traditional belief that LTM is stable over time and resistant to disruption [2, 11–14].

Once formed, the maintenance (or decay) of these memories is dependent upon two neurological processes:

- Memory extinction [15]
- Memory reconsolidation [2]

Memory extinction is a neurological process in which a conditioned stimulus (CS) is repeatedly presented in the absence of the unconditioned stimulus (US), and this eventually leads to a progressive reduction in the expression of the memories such as the fear memories in PTSD or traumatic psychosis. On the other hand, memory reconsolidation is another neurological process in which the retrieval of a previously consolidated memory returns to a labile state after retrieval and is consolidated again (that's why the name is reconsolidation). Thus, in this process of reconsolidation, *the memories that become labile* (rather than stable) *provide a window of opportunity for changing them through interventions.* Reconsolidation is conceptualized as relearning that results in new or updated memories, whereas extinction is a process that involves blocking the original (old) memories by the extinction memory trace [12]. Both memory consolidation and reconsolidation require protein synthesis in the neurons [16]. These findings on reconsolidation fit with the behavioral evidence that retrieved memory is not a carbon copy of the initial memories (primary and secondary memories) because they are updated during the retrieval process.

2.3 Two Different Memory Systems (Verbal and Non-verbal) in Traumatic Memories

According to DSM-5 and ICD-11, the intrusive memories (flashbacks) are categorized under the intrusion symptoms cluster in the diagnosis of PTSD. Among the phenomena in PTSD that need further explanation are the different types of memories observed in this condition, specifically the difference between intrusive memories (flashbacks) and normal autobiographical memory (that we use in everyday life for remembering ordinary past events, the memory of the self which provides us with a sense of identity and continuity). Intrusive memories are fairly common following traumatic experiences, and although in the vast majority of cases they resolve spontaneously, in individuals who develop PTSD or traumatic psychosis they remain ingrained in different brain areas that are involved in the processing of trauma memories (TMs) as discussed in detail later in this chapter.

In the brain, the verbal and non-verbal information are processed separately. The inputs that enter the short-term memory (also called primary memory) are routed through separate locations in the brain depending on whether they are verbal or non-verbal information. For example, the verbal input is attended to and processed in the brain's "phonological loop," whereas the visual input (a non-verbal information) is processed in the brain's "visuospatial sketchpad." From these two different locations, the information is encoded (transferred) to long-term memory. The emotionally salient experiences such as the traumatic memories or the fear memories are stored in the brain as the *emotional memories*. These memories can be positive or negative, but the negative ones such as the traumatic memories have much stronger impact due to their survival value for the individual and the species. The two systems in the brain that store these traumatic memories are known as the Dual Memory Representation (DMR) system which includes the verbal and non-verbal systems [17, 18]. The non-verbal system (also called as the *situationally accessible memory* (SAM) or the sensory-motor system or simply the *sensory memory*) is regarded as evolutionarily primitive, whereas the verbally accessible memory system (VAM) is much more complex and involves the higher order episodic/contextual declarative memory. The primary memory (short-term memory) is always about the present, is a more faithful record of "actual" events, and uses lot of SAM or non-verbal components. In contrast, the secondary or long-term memory belongs to the past and is modified based on salience of the information and the contexts in which the events originally occurred and were processed. Compared to the primary memory, the secondary memory is not a carbon copy of the events as they occurred, rather they are full of distortions and memory gaps and also have more VAM components ([19], page 233). In the SAM system, there is little discrimination of detail or context. On the other hand, in the VAM system, the same signals picked up by the sensory organs are passed to the cerebral cortex of the brain (which is evolutionarily much more recent) for their analysis in much more detail. These signals get processed by the hippocampus as well (which works as the chrono-biographer of events to be stored in the brain) and, if sufficiently rehearsed, get transferred to the long-term autobiographical memory store. With respect to the emotionally charged trauma memories, the SAM (non-verbal) involves the five sense organs including touch, smell, sight, hearing, and taste by which messages are transmitted very rapidly to the amygdala, by using the subcortical pathways and bypassing the cortex (otherwise called the amygdalar hijack [10]). The amygdala and its extension orchestrate the fear response, and this transmission route is "quick and dirty" in the sense that information travels rapidly but is only crudely analyzed. This mechanism of creating the emotional memories is more likely to be generalized as they are not analyzed precisely. Once a particular combination of (conditioned) stimuli is associated with a fear response, a low-level pattern matching system will recreate that fear response (conditioned response) when those stimuli are re-encountered. In PTSD, the conditioning and generalization of the fear responses happen rather quickly, and thus although the traumatic event is specific initially, the triggers for the fear responses soon become relatively non-specific. So, even benign triggers can be sufficient to trigger flashbacks and primary emotions like fear and dread. Even though emotional memories created in this way (in limbic and subcortical areas) are quite strong, they can be superseded by new memories (cognitive memories) that involve the higher (cortical) brain areas: thus, effective psychotherapeutic work which can create healing experiences through creating new learnings and new memories can be eventually effective to supersede these pathologically ingrained emotional memories. Brewin [18], in his dual processing model (DMR), argues that trauma memories show a dissociation or disconnect between the non-verbal (sensory-motor) and verbal (the episodic/declarative) memory systems. Based on our ongoing work, we view that such dissociation is seen in trauma associated treatment resistant depression (TRD) and traumatic psychosis as well. This partly explains why ketamine, a glutamate receptor (N-Methyl D-Aspartate, NMDA) antagonist, is therapeutically effective in TRD [20] and PTSD [13, 14, 21] alike.

2.4 Trauma Memories: The Key Players

The main brain areas involved in processing of trauma or fear memories are the prefrontal cortex (PFC), amygdala, hippocampus, and cerebellum. Medial prefrontal cortex reduces fear responses by reducing the amygdalar output. Many patients afflicted with severe trauma early end up having chronic conditions like treatment refractory PTSD, traumatic psychosis, and borderline personality disorder, among others. These are associated with typically reduced volume and hypofunction of the ventromedial PFC (vmPFC, also called as the infra-limbic (IL) cortex) along with increased amygdala activation and hippocampal shrinkage [22–24]. Both dlPFC (dorsolateral prefrontal cortex) and vmPFC are the centers for the executive functions and cognitive-emotional control, respectively, and there is a reciprocal regulatory connection between vmPFC and the amygdala. One highly consistent finding in the PTSD model of mice is the hypoactivity of the infra-limbic (IL) cortex which concurs with other data, such as the finding that stress-induced extinction impairment is associated with dendritic hypotrophy in the infra-limbic cortex [25]. The fear conditioning response in PTSD uses the pathway of the neural circuit involving the amygdala which receives the inputs regarding the conditioned stimuli from thalamic and sensory cortical areas; this converges with already stored inputs regarding the unconditioned stimulus [26]. The three main things that can modify conditioned fear and its responses are extinction, reversal, and regulation of fear [27].

Research finds that larger brains have more flexible stimulus-response connections and therefore can have a wider range of alternative responses to specific environmental cues [28]. In contrast, smaller brain makes people rigid or inflexible in their behavior because smaller brains represent the world at a more concrete level and also much coarser level of resolution because they have fewer cortical columns to devote to each aspect of represented reality. In the aforementioned conditions resulting from severe trauma in early age, specifically, shrinkage of the CA3 (*cornu ammonis*, region 3) area of the hippocampus occurs. The hippocampus is a crucial brain area for memory (both temporal and spatial memories) and is intimately related to one's ability to construe meanings and regulate emotions: this explains why these people are more reactive and impulsive in nature, are often paranoid, and have pathological distorted views of reality which can result in psychosis. In addition, damage to the dentate gyrus which is one of the very few brain areas that have the ability to regenerate [29] limits new cell production, which in turn may hinder the process of encoding new, differentiated memory patterns [30] and thus impairs new learning. In addition to this, hippocampus is the chronographer of memory; many of these people lose the ability to distinguish between the past and present experiences [31] which explains the reliving symptoms cluster in PTSD. Similarly, the hyperactive amygdala increases encoding of the emotions linked to traumatic memories and makes them more ingrained into the brain and thus more difficult to change [4].

The key players in the brain that process the traumatic memories are amygdala (the "fear center"), the medial prefrontal cortex (mPFC, the "Me Center" or the "self-referencing center"), and the striatum along with cerebellum (both work as the habit- and conditioning-center) [32]. Below is a description of their roles in traumatic memories:

(a) Amygdala (*the fear center*): Integrity of the amygdala is crucial for acquisition and expression of conditioned fear in PTSD: increased amygdalar activation is seen during acquisition or expression of fear, and a reduction of amygdalar activity occurs during the fear extinction or when interventions to regulate the fear are applied. Fear conditioning potentiates the tone responses of neurons in the basolateral amygdala (BLA, the main input pathway to amygdala), which excite the neurons in the central nucleus (Ce) of the amygdala that constitutes the main output pathway from amygdala to brain stem and the autonomic system including the hypothalamic areas, all of which mediate the fear responses such as freezing and startle potentiation. Medial prefrontal cortex prestimulation dramatically reduced the responsiveness of the central nucleus (Ce) output neurons to inputs from the insular cortex and basolateral amygdala (BLA, the main input pathway to amygdala). BLA sends glutamatergic projections to the central nucleus (Ce), and Ce is the main source of amygdala outputs to the brain stem and hypothalamic sites that mediate the behavioral and autonomic correlates of fear.
(b) Medial PFC (mPFC, the *Me Center*): This is a key neural hub in the neurocircuitry model of PTSD. The mPFC is rightly called as the "Me Center" or the "Self-Referencing Center" of the brain because it is deeply involved in building one's notion of self and also plays an important role in self-reflection, empathy, and mentalization (i.e., ability to infer other people's state of mind). The mPFC has two parts: the first part is the ventromedial PFC (vmPFC) which is involved in processing information related to us and people that we view as similar to us and often activated when we take things too personally and hence called as the "unhelpful part" of the MPFC. The second part is the dorsomedial prefrontal cortex (dmPFC) which is involved in processing information related to people we perceive as being *dissimilar* from us and is involved in feeling empathy, especially for people who we perceive of as not being like us and also helps in maintaining social connections.

    The mPFC has robust projections to amygdala. Commonly it shows decreased activation during symptom provocation/triggers and plays an essential role in the inhibition of conditioned fear following extinction [33]. Dorsal part of medial PFC (pre-limbic cortex) reduces fear during extinction, whereas it's ventral part (the ventromedial PFC, vmPFC or infra-limbic cortex/IL) mediates extinction learning and recall by stimulating the inhibitory cells in the amygdala (mostly the GABAergic neurons in its intercalated (ITC) cells which receive a robust projection from mPFC and inhibit the output neurons of amygdala so that fear response is dampened). This leads to arrest of the generation of defense response in response to trauma-related triggers. The vmPFC activation becomes increased in response to the presentation of the CS+ compared with CS during acquisition, followed by a reversal of these responses. In contrast, the lateral region of the ventral PFC is a key structure in reversal of Pavlovian fear conditioning. The mPFC inhibits conditioned fear via feedforward inhibition of Ce output neurons of amygdala. Infra-limbic region of the mPFC appears to be essential for recall of extinction memory, because rats with lesions of IL act as if they never received extinction training. Stimulation of mPFC (as happens in meditation) prevents blood pressure increases induced by exposure to conditioned tones or electrical stimulation of the amygdala.

(c) Cerebellar vermis: It plays a role in fear conditioning consolidation: considering the known role of cerebellum in procedural learning and implicit memory, this finding is not surprising.

2.5 The Newer Cognitive Models of PTSD

Cognitive models of post-traumatic stress disorder (PTSD) developed by Ehlers and Clark [34] and The Emotional Processing Theory by Foa and Kozak [35] have made contributions to the development of efficacious treatments for PTSD. However, these models preceded the rich, contemporary evidence base around the latest neurobiological aspects of PTSD, especially the huge body of memory reconsolidation (and memory extinction) research that has accumulated since 2000. These earlier models have relied on what is now regarded as equivocal evidence around the characteristics of distress maintaining memories [36].

Two more recent and notable cognitive models of PTSD that incorporate the newer research on the neurobiology of trauma/fear memories are the *Core Response Network* (CRN) model and the *Dual Memory Representation* (DMR) model, both of which are described below:

(a) *Core Response Network* (CRN) model: Payne et al. [37] have given substantial considerations to the neurobiological correlates which would explain three of four symptom clusters of PTSD. This theoretical model of trauma explicitly references many of the neurobiological findings mentioned above, specifically the dysfunctionality of the *Core Response Network (CRN).* The CRN consists of the autonomic system (hypothalamus), limbic emotional system (amygdala, hippocampus, and septal region), the emotional motor system (basal ganglia, red nucleus, and periaqueductal grey), and reticular arousal system. In terms of autonomic responses, the traumatic experiences are the result of overactive sympathetic system and underactive parasympathetic system. Per the CRN model, the traumatic situations are responded quickly at a subcortical level, recruiting the autonomic and limbic systems *while leaving the higher cortical regions disengaged.* Of note, the CRN model although explain three of four symptom clusters, does not yet account for re-experiencing and intrusive symptoms and is still accumulating empirical verification.

(b) *The Dual Memory Representation* (DMR) model: Brewin's DMR model [18] mentioned above is deeply rooted in contemporary neurobiological trauma research and does account for intrusive symptoms. Ordinarily, sensory and contextual memory are tightly entwined, and the sensory memory can be retrieved with the assistance of the contextual memory [38]. As mentioned before, the sensory memory (SAM) belongs to more of the primary memory database and involves non-verbal aspects and thus involves more of subcortical areas, whereas the episodic or contextual declarative memory involves verbal parts of the memory and belongs to subsequent orders (secondary, tertiary, etc.) of memory database ([19], page 232–233). During a traumatic incident, diffuse peritraumatic neurobiological networks are activated to capture sensory and motor elements. These networks prioritize sensory-motor mobilization (or catatonic immobilization) against the perceived threat. In susceptible individuals, this can result in the poor integration of diverse perceptual or sensory-motor memories with autobiographical or episodic memory systems [18, 39]. Diffuse processing generates poorly contextualized, fragmented memories. These memories are difficult to control via semantic retrieval or verbal memory systems voluntarily. Instead, SAMs are triggered by traumatic incident specific internal and external sensory cues, and these memories are responsible for arousal maintenance. DMR suggests that these two forms of memory will become dissociated under conditions of extreme emotion, in conjunction with downregulation of the hippocampal system or a dissociative response [38]. Brewin has also cited evidence in support of the temporary nature of sensory memories, and described that exposure (extinction)-based approaches are effective for processing these troubling sensory memories. This is in contrast to episodic (verbal) memories which are strengthened through rehearsal.

2.6 Clinical Relevance of These Findings

As shown in many mice models [26] and more recently also in humans, our ability to extinguish fear/painful memories is known to involve a working connection and coordinated effort between two brain regions: the amygdala and the prefrontal cortex. This has been demonstrated more elegantly by using the optogenetic stimulation technology in rodent models. The experimental control afforded by rodent models, combined with the greater capacity for making precise delineation of neural systems, molecules, and genes in rodents compared with humans, makes them an essential compliment to human studies of traumata and their sequelae like PTSD. The optogenetic technology involves controlling the specific neurons and the resulting animal behavior by using stimulation of neurons by light. This allows to know the precise connection between the two brain regions in real time and provides a more accurate correlation between neuronal activity and behavior. A recent review by researchers at the National Institutes of Health [25] points out that disrupting the amygdala-prefrontal cortex connection resulted in memory extinction failure, i.e., it prevented the mice from overcoming the fear response brought out by a benign trigger for which the mice were conditioned earlier due to repeated exposure. They also found that the opposite is true—that stimulating the circuit results in increased extinction of fearful memories. Another study has similar findings [33]. Given the similarities in fear circuitry between rodents and humans, these new findings inform us that new therapeutic approaches including manipulation of these fear circuitry by pharmacological agents (ketamine, D-cycloserine (DCS), propranolol, etc.) or optogenetic stimulation can have important treatment implications for the chronic and often difficult-to-treat conditions like PTSD. Also, the use of cognitive interventions leads to not only reduction of amygdalar activity but also activation of important regulatory brain areas such as the dorsolateral PFC (dlPFC) and ventromedial PFC (vmPFC, otherwise called as the infra-limbic cortex/IL) as measured by the BOLD (blood oxygen level dependent) signals in functional MRI (fMRI) [26]. This provides a rationale for use of brain stimulation therapy such as repetitive transcranial magnetic stimulation (rTMS) for patients with refractory PTSD. Using rTMS and TIMBER concurrently during the rTMS therapy session, Pradhan et al. [40] have successfully treated four patients with refractory PTSD. This updated review provides one of the bases for therapeutic manipulation of the pathological memories, as done in TIMBER psychotherapy which can be used as a standalone therapy or in combination with other cutting-edge treatment modalities such as subanesthetic infusion of ketamine [13, 14] or with brain stimulation therapy using rTMS [41].

The deep connections between the stress and multiple memory systems deserve a special mention. Stress influences the quality of memories formed [42]. Among the multiple memory systems, the important ones are the *explicit* or *declarative memory* which is hippocampus dependent, and the *implicit* or h*abitual* memories which are based on the striatum (and cerebellum). Under stress, *the hippocampal-based declarative memory is impaired, whereas the striatal-based implicit or habitual memories are unaffected or even boosted* [42]. *Thus, stress causes an increase in habitual behavior (striatal mediated) at the expense of goal-directed behavior (prefrontal cortex mediated).* In vulnerable individuals like the clients afflicted with trauma, these stress-induced shifts might influence the chronicity of the symptoms and thus treatment outcomes.

Also, in the context of chronic PTSD, the updated research findings on the two memory systems (verbal and sensorimotor/non-verbal) involved in trauma mentioned above are quite important because most of the existing talk therapies target the verbal/declarative memories which leaves the non-verbal components unaddressed. For comprehensive care, therapies need to address both verbal and non-verbal components of the trauma memories. The *Arousal Response to Trauma Memories Reactivation* (ART-MR, [13]) a trauma specific scale developed by Pradhan and Gray takes into accounts for both the verbal and non-verbal aspects of expression of trauma memories and can serve as a useful scale in this regard. Also use of this scale helps in keeping the exposure during therapy controlled and not overflood the patients so that secondary traumatization in therapy settings are prevented of the ART-MR scores during exposure sessions are kept below 30 (maximum score in the 11-item ART-MR scale is 55).

With respect to the future novel interventions for trauma-afflicted patients, role of brain-derived neurotrophic factor (BDNF) deserves special mention. BDNF promotes the proliferation, survival, and differentiation of neurons and also plays a role in abnormal fear and memory extinction. It has been found that patients who suffer from traumatic events have a lower BDNF levels in serum. Thus, genes involved in regulation of the BDNF are currently the genes of interest for PTSD since pathological fear is a central feature of PTSD. This was shown in a study [43] which revealed that the targeted knockdown or inhibition of BDNF-TrkB signaling in the amygdala resulted in loss of fear memory acquisition, and hippocampal deletion of BDNF led to disrupted extinction of fear memory. These results indicate that BDNF is essential for fear memory formation and extinction in multiple cortico-limbic structures and may be a therapeutic target for PTSD.

2.7 Conclusions and Future Directions

Recent research does shed light on the pathogenetic nature of deeply ingrained traumatic memories (TMs) in post-traumatic stress disorder (PTSD), traumatic psychosis, and treatment resistant depression (TRD), especially in the settings of trauma. The disturbed functionality of the neural circuits involved in the processing and expression of the traumatic memories perpetuates the symptoms in these conditions. These are intricately linked to the effects of the contexts in which trauma occurred and also linked to the individual as well as social, environmental, and genetic risk factors, which converge on these neural networks. New translational research strategies are needed to delineate as well as mechanistically tap into the various trajectories involved in the expression of traumatic memories so that more efficacious and evidence-based interventions can be developed and tested reliably [44]. The in-depth understanding of these mechanisms holds the prospect of novel strategies for pharmacology, psychotherapy, gene therapy, and social policy that target and converge on the identified neural circuits and gene targets. A renewed focus on these aspects, therefore, has much to offer for scientists, patients, and therapists alike. These aspects are important to study further with respect to their mechanisms so that novel interventions can be developed that can target the maladaptive memories in the clinical settings for these often difficult-to-treat conditions. Hopefully, this rapidly expanding field that has so far provided many exciting data pertaining will be able to provide meaningful answers in distant future if not too soon.

References

1. Irving J. A prayer for Owen Meany: a novel. 1st ed. New York, NY: William Morrow; 1989.
2. Nader K, Schafe GE, LeDoux JE. Fear memories require protein synthesis in the amygdala for reconsolidation after retrieval. Nature. 2000;406:722–6.
3. Shin LM, Liberzon I. The neurocircuitry of fear, stress and anxiety disorders. Neuropsychopharmacology. 2010;35(2010):169–91.
4. Soeter M, Kindt M. Dissociating response systems. Erasing fear from memory. Neurobiol Learn Mem. 2010;94(1):30–41.
5. Hoge CW, Grossman SH, Auchterlonie JL, Riviere LA, Milliken CS, Wilk JE. PTSD treatment for soldiers after combat deployment: low utilization of mental health care and reasons for dropout. Psychiatr Serv. 2014;65:997–1004.

6. Kessler RC, Chiu WT, Demler O, Merikangas KR, Walters EE. Prevalence, severity, and comorbidity of 12-month DSM- IV disorders in the National Comorbidity Survey Replication. Arch Gen Psychiatry. 2005;62:617–27.
7. Kandel E, et al. Prefrontal cortex, hippo- campus, and the biology of explicit memory storage. Principles of Neural Science. 5th ed. New York, Chicago, San-Francisco: McGraw-Hill Companies, Inc.; 2013.
8. McDermott KB, Roediger HL. Memory (encoding, storage, retrieval). In: Biswas-Diener R, Diener E, editors. Noba textbook series: Psychology. Champaign, IL: DEF publishers; 2019.
9. Tulving E. Are there 256 different kinds of memory? In: Nairne JS, editor. The foundations of remembering: essays in honor of Henry L. Roediger, III. New York: Psychology Press; 2007. p. 39–52.
10. LeDoux JE. Emotion circuits in the brain. Annu Rev Neurosci. 2000;23:155–84.
11. Dudai Y. Reconsolidation: the advantage of being refocused. Curr Opin Neurobiol. 2006;16(2):174–8.
12. Monfils MH, Cowansage KK, Klann E, LeDoux JE. Extinction-reconsolidation boundaries: key to persistent attenuation of fear memories. Science. 2009;324:951–5.
13. Pradhan BK, Wainer IW, Moaddel R, et al. Trauma Interventions using Mindfulness Based Extinction and Reconsolidation (TIMBER) psychotherapy prolong the therapeutic effects of single ketamine infusion on post-traumatic stress disorder and comorbid depression: a pilot randomized, placebo-controlled, cross-over clinical trial. Asia Pac J Clin Trials Nerv Syst Dis. 2017;2(2017):80–90.
14. Pradhan BK, Mitrev L, Moaddel R, Wainer I. D-Serine is a biomarker for clinical response in (R, S)-ketamine treatment of post-traumatic stress disorder and co-morbid depression. Biochim Biophys Acta. 2018a;S1570-9639(18):30035–9.
15. Westbrook RF, Iordanova M, McNally G, Richardson R, Harris JA. Reinstatement of fear to an extinguished conditioned stimulus: two roles for context. J Exp Psychol Anim Behav Process. 2002;28:97–110.
16. Alberini CM. Mechanisms of memory stabilization: are consolidation and reconsolidation similar or distinct processes? Trends Neurosci. 2005;28(1):51–6.
17. Brewin CR. A cognitive neuroscience account of posttraumatic stress disorder and its treatment. Behav Res Ther. 2001;39:373–93.
18. Brewin CR. Re-experiencing traumatic events in PTSD: new avenues in research on intrusive memories and flashbacks. Eur J Psychotraumatol. 2015;6:27180. https://doi.org/10.3402/ejpt.v6.27180.
19. Pradhan BK. Yoga and mindfulness based cognitive therapy: a clinical guide. Switzerland: Springer; 2014.
20. Aan Het Rot M, Zarate CA Jr, Charney DS, Mathew SJ. Ketamine for depression: where do we go from here? Biol Psychiat. 2012;72:537–47.
21. Feder A, Parides MK, Murrough JW, Perez AM, Morgan J, Saxena S, Kirkwood K, aan het Rot M, Lapidus KAB, Wan L-B, Losifescu D, Charney DS. Efficacy of intravenous ketamine for treatment of chronic posttraumatic stress disorder: a randomized clinical trial. JAMA Psychiat. 2014;71:681–8.
22. Cardenas VA, Samuelson K, Lenoci M, Studholme C, Neylan TC, Marmar CR, Schuff N, Weiner MW. Changes in brain anatomy during the course of PTSD. Psychiatry Res. 2011;193(2):93–100.
23. Hull A. Neuroimaging findings in post-traumatic stress disorder: systematic review. Br J Psychiatry. 2002;181:102–10.
24. Teicher MH, Andersen SL, Polcari A, et al. Developmental neurobiology of childhood stress and trauma. Psychiatr Clin North Am. 2002;25:397–426.
25. Holmes A, Singewald N. Individual differences in recovery from traumatic fear. Trends Neurosci. 2013;36(1):23–31.
26. Parsons RG, Ressler KJ. Implications of memory modulation for post-traumatic stress and fear disorders. Nat Neurosci. 2013;16(2):146–53.

27. Schiller D, Monfils MH, Raio CM, Johnson DC, Ledoux JE, Phelps EA. Preventing the return of fear in humans using reconsolidation update mechanisms. Nature. 2010;463:49–53.
28. Tanaka K. Columns for complex visual object features in the inferotemporal cortex: clustering of cells with similar but slightly different stimulus selectivities. Cereb Cortex. 2003;13:90–9.
29. Gaze FH. Neurogenesis in the adult brain. J Neurosci. 2002;22(3):612–3.
30. Kemperman G. Why new neurons? Possible functions for adult hippocampal neurogenesis. J Neurosci. 2002;22:635–8.
31. Diergaarde L, Schoffelmeer ANM, De Vries TJ. Pharmacological manipulation of memory reconsolidation: towards a novel treatment of pathogenic memories. Eur J Pharmacol. 2008;585(2–3):453–7.
32. Pradhan BK, Gogineni RR, Sharma S. Mind, mindfulness, and the social brain: psychobiological understandings and implications. Ind J Social Psychiat. 2018b;34(4):313–22.
33. Quirk GJ, Likhtik E, Pelletier JG, Pare D. Stimulation of medial prefrontal cortex decreases the responsiveness of central amygdala output neurons. J Neurosci. 2003;23(25):8800–7.
34. Ehlers A, Clark DM. A cognitive model of posttraumatic stress disorder. Behav Res Ther. 2000;38:319–45.
35. Foa EB, Kozak MJ. Emotional processing of fear: exposure to corrective information. Psychol Bull. 1986;99(1):20–35.
36. Lancaster SC, Rodriguez BF, Weston V. Path analytic examination of the cognitive model of PTSD. Behav Res Ther. 2011;49(3):194–201.
37. Payne P, Levine PA, Crane-Godreau MA. Somatic experiencing: using interoception and proprioception of core elements of trauma therapy. Front Psychol. 2015;6:93. https://doi.org/10.3389/fpsyg.2015.00093.
38. Brewin CR, Burgess N. Contextualisation in the revised dual representation theory of PTSD: A response to Pearson and colleagues. J Behav Ther Exp Psychiat. 2013;45(1):217–9.
39. Brewin C. Episodic memory, perceptual memory, and their interaction: foundations for a theory of posttraumatic stress disorder. Psychol Bull. 2014;140:69–97.
40. Pradhan BK, Biswal B, Elman I. (2016–2019, unpublished study). Combining brain stimulation (rTMS) and mindfulness therapy (TIMBER) for chronic PTSD: Pilot data on 3 patients.
41. Pradhan BK, Elman I. (2017). Combining brain stimulation (rTMS) and mindfulness therapy (TIMBER) for chronic PTSD: Pilot data on 3 patients.
42. Fink G. Stress: neuroendocrinology and neurobiology. In: Handbook of stress, vol. 2. Dan Diego, CA: Academic Press, Elsevier; 2017.
43. Dell'Osso L, Carmassi C, Del Debbio A, Catena Dell'Osso M, Bianchi C, et al. Brain-derived neurotrophic factor plasma levels in patients suffering from post-traumatic stress disorder. Prog Neuro-Psychopharmacol Biol Psychiatry. 2009;33:899–902.
44. Visser RM, Lau-Zhu A, Henson RN, Holmes EA. Multiple memory systems, multiple time points: how science can inform treatment to control the expression of unwanted emotional memories. Phil Trans R Soc B. 2018;373:20170209.

Part II

TIMBER Therapy for PTSD, Depression and Traumatic Psychosis: Methodology, Application and Efficacy

Trauma Interventions Using Mindfulness-Based Extinction and Reconsolidation of Memories (TIMBER)

3

3.1 Introduction

Current pharmacological and psychotherapeutic treatment strategies for chronic post-traumatic stress disorder (PTSD), treatment resistant depression (TRD), and traumatic psychosis are limited in effectiveness, so innovative interventions are urgently needed for patients suffering from these complex conditions. Only about 60% of patients with PTSD respond to the frontline antidepressant (SSRIs) therapy and about 20–30% of them drop out from prolonged exposure therapy [1]. Drop out from exposure therapy (based on *extinction-only mechanism* rather than pairing extinction with reconsolidation) is likely to be related to lack of efficacy, over-flooding, and re-traumatization during therapy [2]. The efficacy of cognitive-behavioral therapy (CBT) interventions for PTSD, TRD in trauma settings, and traumatic psychosis and are established but have important limitations not only with respect to techniques but also feasibility and user friendliness. As detailed in Chap. 2, the deeply ingrained emotionally changed traumatic memories (TMs) are the critical factors in maintaining symptoms in these three conditions, but current treatment strategies don't directly or efficiently address them [3, 4]. The result is that there is a risk of either insufficient or uncontrolled activation of the TMs in the treatment settings which may lead to lack of response or more often than not, relapse.

Mindfulness-based cognitive-behavioral therapy is a type of CBT that has been well studied in subjects with treatment resistant depression, both for acute phase and for relapse prevention with demonstrated efficacy [5–7]. This therapy changes the relationship between the individual and their negative thoughts and emotions. Instead of an adversarial relationship of controlling or changing the thoughts, strategies of acceptance and enhanced self-compassion bring about symptom improvement and prevent relapse. TIMBER (*Trauma Interventions* using *Mindfulness-Based Extinction and Reconsolidation* of memories) psychotherapy is a novel, translational, and neurobiologically informed Yoga and mindfulness-based cognitive-behavioral therapy (Y-MBCT, [8]) developed to help bridge some of the existing treatment gaps in PTSD, TRD in trauma settings, and traumatic psychosis. These

B. Pradhan et al., *TIMBER Psychotherapy*,
https://doi.org/10.1007/978-3-030-20648-2_3

three conditions are often a sequelae of trauma and have TMs as the core psychopathology. In the following sections, we elaborate on the components and processes involved in TIMBER, followed by demonstration of the mechanism of action of this therapy. We then guide the reader through the process of delivering TIMBER followed by the evidence base.

3.2 Need to Pair the Extinction with Reconsolidation as Done in TIMBER

Targeting to modify the emotionally charged traumatic memories, TIMBER, as its name suggests, uses a balanced combination of two main memory modifying mechanisms, i.e., *memory extinction* and *memory reconsolidation*. Trauma memory extinction is the gradual diminishing of an emotionally charged conditioned response over time as a person learns to uncouple a response from a stimulus during repeated exposure. Trauma memory reconsolidation is retrieval of the traumatic memories to strengthen, add, or remove information and then update them in a new setting or context [9]. TIMBER capitalizes on the fact that controlled reactivation of TMs makes them labile and thus prone to change (reconsolidation) but do not overflood or re-traumatize the patient. Most of the current therapies to treat trauma-related symptoms are based on memory extinction-only mechanism (e.g., prolonged exposure therapy) and have important limitations in their effectiveness. Some of these limitations include *spontaneous recovery* of the extinguished memories, *renewal* of these memories, their *reinstatement*, and their *rapid reacquisition* in a new context/setting of trauma, thus leading to insufficient recovery or eventual relapse [10, 11]. In contrast, memory reconsolidation is a newer concept that attempts to modify the existing and pathologically ingrained traumatic memories resulting in the formation of *new memories* and, thereby, *offering a distinct advantage over extinction-only approaches.* Recent work on memory shows that extinction should be paired with reconsolidation in order to build the skills as well as the resilience in dealing with the traumatic memories and the conditions resulting from them [12]. Devising novel interventions that utilize concepts from both memory extinction and reconsolidation mechanisms helps us to better deal with the traumatic memories as already discussed in Chap. 2.

As a Yoga and mindfulness-based cognitive therapy (Y-MBCT) method, TIMBER has been specifically designed for treatment of chronic PTSD, treatment resistant depression, and traumatic psychosis and technically belongs to the emerging category of *third wave* CBT interventions [13]. The psychological processes that make individuals prone to relapse in chronic PTSD, treatment resistant depression, and traumatic psychosis are also likely to be active in perpetuating their symptoms in these conditions [5, 14]. These processes are governed by the deeply ingrained TMs, thus making TIMBER effective for these three conditions. TIMBER is a *targeted, time limited, and translational (3Ts)* mindfulness-based cognitive-behavioral therapy (CBT). Its targeted nature is already explained, and its time-limited nature (8–12 sessions done over a period of 4–6 months) has been elaborated later. It is translational because it incorporates the basic science knowledge (such as neurobiological mechanisms of trauma memory processing, biological markers of response to treatment, etc.) into its methodology and applies them pragmatically into clinical settings.

3.3 Need to Combine Many Therapeutic Components as Done in TIMBER

Yoga and mindfulness-based interventions have been studied in several psychiatric conditions such as PTSD, anxiety disorders, major depressive disorder, and psychotic disorders ([5, 15, 16]). However, there are several limitations in the way some of these concepts from ancient Eastern practices have been incorporated into the Western science. Yoga and meditation interventions are heterogeneous, involve many different components, and are often not being used in a standardized manner. There are a large number of mysteries and distorted views surrounding Yoga and meditation with a lack of clarity as to what they mean in practice, especially in clinical settings. In addition, there has been a piecemeal and non-targeted or non-specific use of Yoga and meditation intervention. For example, Yoga is largely understood as a physical or postural technique and meditation as a breathing technique. This kind of dichotomous view and fragmented use of Yoga and meditation restrict their scope as well as utility and may come in the way of the integration of the body and mind. This is illustrated in an interesting review of Vietnam veterans suffering from PTSD [16] in which the authors found that although using the physical aspects of Yoga such as physical postures (Sanskrit: *asana*) did indeed reduce some symptoms of comorbid depression, they had no impact on the hyperarousal symptoms, panic, or anger outbursts until meditation interventions including meditative breathing methods (Sanskrit: *pranayama*) and focused attention meditation were added. Thus, Yoga and meditation interventions are more effective when these multiple components are understood and used in combined, synergistic, and targeted ways. This elaborative and integrated approach is in accordance with the ancient Indian scheme of the *Eight-limbed Yoga of Patanjali* (Sanskrit: *Ashtanga Yoga*, [17]), or the *Noble Eightfold Path of the Buddha* (Pali. *Atthangika Magga,* [18]) as they were proposed originally [8]. Other literature [15, 19] indicates that integrated use of multiple components of Yoga rather than their use in isolation or piecemeal, as individual components, is more effective in clinical trials. The non-standardized and non-specific approaches pose significant challenges in research when one tries to evaluate the comparative efficacy of the Yoga or meditation interventions across studies [15].

TIMBER involves a broad array of many psychotherapeutic components which can be categorized under two main groups: (a) *standardized Yoga and meditation protocols,* and (b) two main CBT methods which are (1) *mindfulness-based graded exposure therapy* (MB-GET, [8, 20], illustrated in Fig. 3.1) and (2) *cognitive reformulation and reprocessing* of the traumatic memories in less emotional ways by use of the mindful state. These three aspects are described briefly below and elaborated in later parts of this chapter:

1. *Training on the standardized Yoga and meditation protocols:* This forms the first step in TIMBER therapy before conducting the graded exposure (MB-GET). This step helps the client to regain the state of mind (the mindful state) necessary to observe the trauma symptoms and the life problems more neutrally or in a less reactive manner rather than being flooded by or habitually repeating them with-

out control. The mindful state (which is *simultaneously alert, calm, and detached/non-reactive*), once attained, brings more focus and attentional reorientation so that the client can engage in non-judgmental self-observation of their *thoughts, feelings, (traumatic) memories, sensations, and impulses/behaviors* (this is called the Buddha's *five factors model of human experience*, [8]) rather than habitually indulging in them in repetitive and emotionally charged manner.

2. *The mindfulness-based graded exposure therapy* (MB-GET, Fig. 3.1): this is the second step in TIMBER which involves the following:
    (a) Behavior analysis (antecedent, behavior, and consequences: the *ABC paradigm*) of the trauma-related avoidance and hyperarousal symptoms.
    (b) Using the trauma-triggers list and building up the anxiety pyramid in a hierarchical order from 10 to 100% subjective units of distress (SUD).

Mindfulness Based Graded Exposure Therapy (MB-GET©: Pradhan, B.K., 2013)

Name: **Date of Birth** **Highest level of Education:** **Date:**

MB-GET© is a group of highly individualized & scientifically proven therapies for refractory psychiatric symptoms, designed by Dr. Pradhan & used at Cooper University Hospital. This will involve first building a **PYRAMID of anxiety/stress triggers** in your daily life & then establishing home practice sessions for handling these triggers so that their progression to full blown episodes is prevented. This requires your own efforts & guidance from Dr. Pradhan/his associates. The figure below illustrates these points. MB-GET interventions are strategically designed for your body and mind by use of calming breathing meditations, mindful awareness training and meditative life style (*Middle Way*). **The first step in designing your personalized therapy program is to build the TRIGGER PYRAMID** by doing a thorough analysis of situations in your daily life that trigger your anxiety/stress & force you to avoid these situations. Once you're trained, you'll gradually expose yourself to these triggers: *first with help of Dr. Pradhan & his associates in the session, and then on your own during home practice.* Any discomfort that may arise can be handled by practicing the **symptom specific techniques which can be used alone or with meds. The complete treatment course typically involves mindfulness training over about 6-12 sessions (with therapist) along with symptom specific HOME PRACTICE (on your own).**

[illegible] **identify 3 main trigger situations & build the TRIGGER PYRAMID.** **Below, please list *specific persons, objects, situations in daily life* that trigger your outbursts or symptoms or episodes.**	**Anxiety/fear/ distress caused by the triggers (10-100%)**	**Please describe your behaviors, feelings & thoughts in these situations**
1.	100% level	
2.		
3.	30-40% level will be your start point	
In the above situations, what are the first symptoms in **BODY** (hyperventilation, butterfly in stomach, fidgety, feeling warm etc.):		
In your daily life, please describe the **SEQUENCE of progression of symptoms in a typical full blown *episode*** *of panic/anxiety/anger/sadness:*		

Mindfulness Toolbox:

- ▯ **BREATHING *MEDITATIONS* to ▯ anger, flashbacks, panic, sadness, physical symptoms, insomnia, dissociative symptoms**
- ▯ **STOPP technique: ROUTINE practice, Morning & Night (60-70 breaths) + AS NEEDED practice, 10-15 breaths each time**
- ▯ ***The Middle Way:* Not to engage in extremes**
- ▯ **Five Factor Model of the Mind: To induce Detachment from symptoms or thoughts or feelings etc.**
- ▯ **Practice Log & Flash Cards for mindfulness practice**

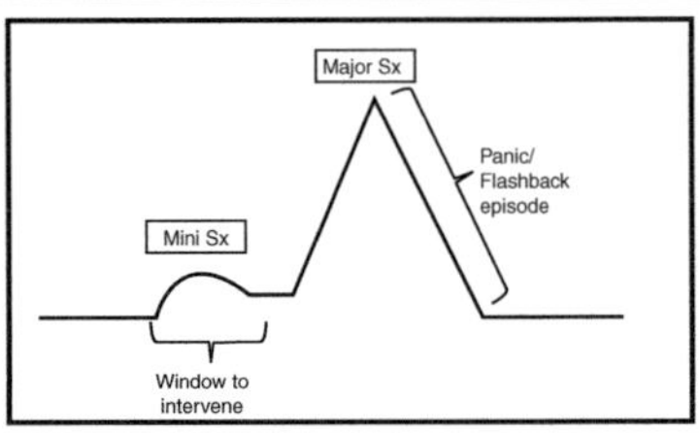

SEQUENCE to CONTROL SYMPTOMS

REFERENCES: 1-*Yoga & Mindfulness Based Cognitive Therapy: A Clinical Guide* (Pradhan, B.K., 2014; Springer Publishers)
2-Dr. Pradhan's YouTube video: *http://youtu.be/pvHDCZ5D7Xk*

Fig. 3.1 Scheme of the mindfulness-based graded exposure therapy (MB-GET)

(c) First inducing the mindfulness state in the client followed by therapist-assisted exposure of the client in graded manner (10–100% SUD) over 5–8 sessions as tolerated. That's why the name is mindfulness-based graded exposure therapy (MB-GET).

MB-GET involves *increased awareness but less reactivity* to both the symptoms and their precursors (antecedents or trauma triggers) which is *exactly opposite to the typical pattern of dissociation* (less awareness) *and hyperarousals* seen in clients afflicted with trauma. The act of consciously, purposefully, and calmly paying attention to the symptoms of trauma, their antecedents, and consequences as done in MB-GET is truly a contemplation and is r*esponsive* rather than reactive. This contemplation makes these symptoms more objective targets of reflection and detached observation rather than an intolerable source of subjective anger, anxiety, frustration, and dysphoria. Also MB-GET prevents overflooding and promotes client engagement. We notice that once trained in the standardized Yoga and meditation protocols to recreate a mindfulness state, in TIMBER, often clients are more relaxed and willing to start the exposure with 30–40% SUD, whereas in many other therapy protocols (such as systematic desensitization) often clients start reluctantly with a lower level (around 5–10%) SUD level [21].

3. *Non-reactive cognitive reprocessing of the traumatic memories*: this forms the third step in TIMBER and involves conducting the formal CBT using the thought record and coping skills enhancement, etc. In this step, the client first practices meditation with the therapist in the session, and once mindful state is established, cognitive restructuring, reformulation, and reappraaisal of the traumatic memories are done in a non-reactive or calm way. This *decreases the threat value of the traumatic memories further* which have been already lessened during the graded exposure done in the previous step (memory extinction component of TIMBER) and *provides new meanings to them* which are less threatening and more open-minded with more alternative (often healthy) thoughts and explanations incorporated in them. Thus, in this step, *the memories are updated and rewritten with new meanings* originating from this new, calm, and non-threatening context. This is the memory reconsolidation component of TIMBER.

Use of multiple components in a synergistic manner probably explains the superior efficacy of TIMBER as seen in the placebo-controlled randomized studies [14, 22]. The translational concepts and design and the customized and targeted interventions done in TIMBER are aimed to cause a paradigm shift in trauma therapy so that treatment outcomes can be improved.

The following are the five main goals of TIMBER psychotherapy:

1. Creating and maintaining a meditative state of mind that is *calm, alert, and non-reactive*. This state prevents flooding and re-traumatization that is seen in some other exposure-based treatment approaches.
2. Improvement in core symptoms and associated symptoms of PTSD or TRD or psychosis.

3. Improvement in avoidance behaviors related to trauma.
4. Improvement in functioning of the individual.
5. Improvements in quality of life.

3.4 Mechanism of TIMBER Psychotherapy

TIMBER is founded on the simple yet elegant fact that the extinction of the emotionally charged traumatic memories (TMs), the reconsolidation of the calming memories generated through meditation, and detached or non-reactive reformulation of these TMs can occur best in a mindful state. The *mindful state* has *three characteristics*: *it is alert, it is calm, and it is non-reactive and not jumpy or emotionally unsettling. Thus, if a person's state of mind at any time is simultaneously alert, relaxed, and detached (non-reactive), a state of mindfulness can be said to have attained in that person at that moment.* In TIMBER, the process of extinction of trauma memories, reconsolidation of calming memories, and detached reformulation of pathological memories using the mindful state allow the amelioration of the symptoms of chronic PTSD, treatment resistant depression, and traumatic psychosis. The unique and standardized methodology of TIMBER keeps the trauma memory retrieval controlled and the hyperarousal symptoms not too overwhelming so that it does not cause overflooding and re-traumatization for clients that is seen more often than not in some other exposure-based treatment approaches.

3.5 Unique Features of TIMBER When Dealing with Trauma Memories

1. TIMBER uses controlled reactivation of trauma memories for effective reconsolidation rather than over-flooding by using four key aspects: (a) use of the *Arousal Response to Trauma Memory Reactivation (*ART-MR), a standardized scale specifically designed for this purpose (details are presented in Chap. 4); (b) use of the brief narrative of the index trauma that takes into account both the verbal and non-verbal aspects of the expressions of traumatic memories; (c) the unique methodology of the mindfulness-based graded exposure therapy (MB-GET, [8, 20]) that not only builds the skills before exposure but also makes the exposure graded as well as sequential, i.e., imaginative exposure first followed by when client is ready, in vivo exposure; and (d) customization and individualization of the interventions by use of the mindfulness profile of the client generated by use of *Assessment Scale for Mindfulness Interventions (ASMI), a scale specifically designed for this purpose.*
2. TIMBER uses two mechanisms (extinction and reconsolidation) in a balanced combination for changing the expression of traumatic memories. Of note, most contemporary trauma treatments use extinction-only approach which has limitations in the form of context dependency, and just suppressing the memories rather than updating them can lead to quicker relapse in new settings of trauma and related triggers.

3. TIMBER has two versions: Full TIMBER and mini-TIMBER (STOPP module, Fig. 3.2).
   (a) Full *TIMBER*: This is the longer version (20–40 min therapy session) which is therapist assisted and focuses on the calming memory reconsolidation and trauma memory extinction by first creating the mindful state and then using the mindfulness-based graded exposure therapy (MB-GET) interventions, respectively.
   (b) Mini-*TIMBER* (STOPP module, Fig. 3.2): This is the shorter version (5-min session) that is ideally suited for home practice by the client once the skills have been established by use of the Full TIMBER. The mini-TIMBER or the STOPP module of mindfulness is Pradhan's behavioral adaptation of the *Middle Way* philosophy of mindfulness traditions, which he has successfully applied in clinical situations within the age range of 6–80 years [22]. STOPP is an acronym for *S*tress, *T*hree (or *T*en or *T*wenty) breaths, *O*bserve, *P*ractice and *P*rogress. Mini-TIMBER specifically helps the clients to quickly de-escalate the arousal symptoms as they arise spontaneously in their daily life situations in response to trauma-related cues/triggers.

Thus, by the ongoing use of both Full TIMBER and mini-TIMBER, subsequent calm and detached reappraisal of expressions of trauma memories is achieved, and new learning becomes possible in the clients to assist in their recovery.

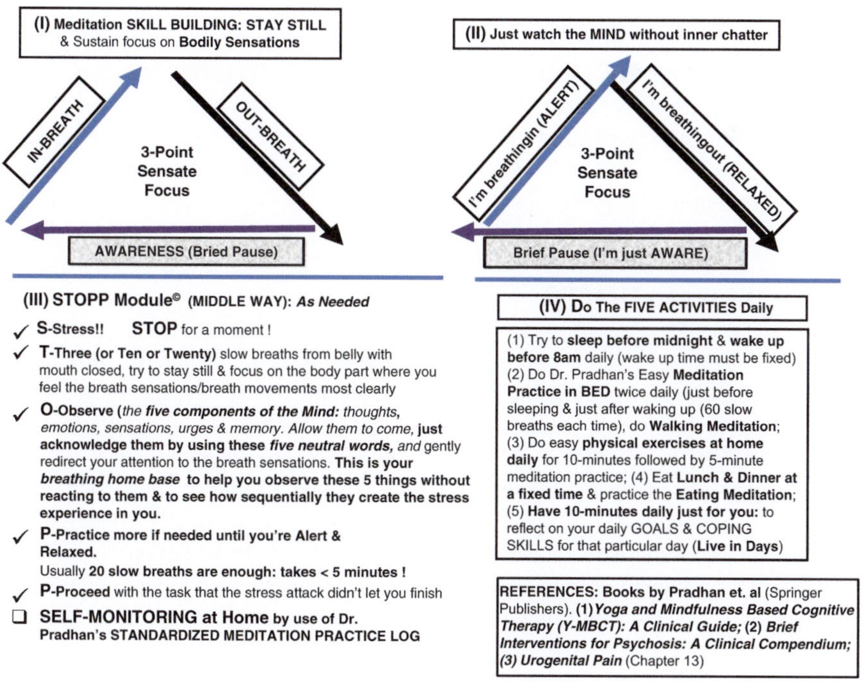

Fig. 3.2 Standardized Yoga and meditation training in TIMBER in four steps

3.6 Delivery of TIMBER

Interventions in TIMBER psychotherapy are utilized in a user friendly self-help format to target and attempt to change the emotionally charged trauma memories and their expressions in an individuals' daily life. TIMBER teaches clients to access the mindful state (calm, alert, and non-reactive state) in the session with the therapist's help. Subsequently this state can be achieved by the client at home using the home practice module and eventually generalizing to other real-life situations. The calm state allows clients to access pathological memories without reacting to them. Thus, they are reconsolidated (as new memories) without the associated emotional distress. Cultivation of this mindful state allows not only detached or neutral reappraisal (extinction) of the traumatic memories and their expressions but also allows reconsolidation of calming memories and facilitates more therapeutic work using CBT interventions (such as mindfulness-based graded exposure therapy, MB-GET, and cognitive restructuring).

The meditation skills that help to access the mindful state when used as a daily routine (more than 10 min, at least twice daily) in practice sessions as well as when needed (de novo, short, less than 5 min) reduce the baseline hyperarousal and gradually make the client achieve the mindful state. This allows the individual to achieve the basic state needed to apply the TIMBER interventions in trauma-specific ways.

"Mindful state" is a state where there is less psychological distress; the individual is self-assured and self-controlled and feels resilient. Using the mindful state to experience the trauma memories in a clam manner (extinction of the emotional memories), the process of detached reformulation of those, and the reconsolidation of calming memories allow individuals to ameliorate the symptoms of PTSD, treatment resistant depression, and traumatic psychosis. The ongoing practice over a period of 3–6 months is shown to help maintain a more sustained mindful state that correlates with improved role functioning and enhanced neuroplasticity as seen in our recent studies that used TIMBER with ketamine infusion [14, 22] and brain stimulation treatment (rTMS) [23].

3.7 Stages in TIMBER

TIMBER uses a two-staged approach: the initial *wellness model* and the subsequent *illness-/disorder-specific* model. TIMBER first ensures skill building in the client and caregivers by formal training in Yoga and meditation by the *Standardized Meditation Program (StaMP)* which forms its *wellness component*. This training takes 2–3 sessions, done at a frequency of once a week, 30-min duration each. After these skills are achieved, it specifically focuses on systematically changing the expressions of traumatic memories in the client's daily life by use of two main CBT methods which constitute its *illness- or disorder-specific component*. These two CBT methods are the mindfulness-based graded exposure therapy (MB-GET, [8, 20]) and cognitive reprocessing of the traumatic memories after the mindful state has been achieved. Both wellness and the illness models initially use the *therapist-assisted training* of client (as well as caregivers and therapist, if appropriate) followed by home practice to enhance meditation skills and reduce stress in daily life situations afflicted with trauma. Once the meditation skill is built, and clients are able to recreate the mindful state (i.e., they are alert, calm, and not that much reactive/hyperaroused), they are trained in the *illness-/disorder-specific* model that modifies the expression of trauma memories in a targeted way, using a combination of mindfulness-based graded exposure therapy (MB-GET) and cognitive reprocessing in detached reappraisal mode using standardized meditation protocols.

To target the trauma memories, TIMBER is delivered in two stages:

1. The shorter mini-TIMBER (STOPP module): This takes 5–10 min to apply and uses calming memory reconsolidation format.
2. The longer full-TIMBER that takes 20–40 min to apply and uses the trauma memory extinction format.

To be able to assess and deliver interventions objectively and in targeted ways, TIMBER uses two specific scales:

1. *Assessment Scale for Mindfulness Interventions* (ASMI).
2. *Arousal Response to Trauma Memory Reactivation* (ART-MR) [8]

The wellness component of TIMBER is aimed at stress reduction and improving coping in the clients and their significant others, while the illness component targets the trauma memories and their expressions. In TIMBER, the experiential aspects and fidelity of its application are enhanced by the therapist practicing with the clients during the therapy sessions. In addition to enhancing empathy, this enhances the therapist's expertise in applying the model, as well as helps with therapist's own stress.

3.8 The Nuts and Bolts in Applying TIMBER Therapy

TIMBER consists of 8–12 structured, skills-based, weekly individual therapy sessions (which can be used in the group setting as well), each lasting for 20–40 min. After the client is trained in the course of TIMBER, there can be 3–4 booster sessions administered at a frequency that can be collaboratively decided by the client and therapist. TIMBER is delivered first in a therapist-assisted exposure format, followed later by the home practice sessions using self-exposure format. As detailed below, *TIMBER uses elements of both cognitive-behavioral therapy (CBT) and mindfulness-based cognitive therapy (MBCT) in addition to teaching clients a family of other interventions*. These include formal sitting meditations (both focused attention type and detachment/open monitoring types) mixed with Yogic postures, breathing practices, informal mindfulness practices (e.g., mindfulness of everyday activities like walking meditation, eating meditation, etc.), and the mindfulness-based graded exposure therapy (MB-GET, a type of CBT, [24]).

The difference between CBT, MBCT, and TIMBER is illustrated. For example, in case of a depressed individual who thinks, "I am a bad and defective person." CBT therapist might challenge the validity of this negative automatic thought and then attempt to change this thought pattern. On the other hand, a MBCT therapist teaches clients to de-identify with the thought by simply recognizing that "I am having the thought that I'm a bad and defective person," to realize that thought is not necessarily a fact, and then let go of the thought. In contrast, in TIMBER, unlike in CBT, the therapist at first trains the client on how to change the relationship one has to his or her thoughts as well as other mental experiences including emotions, memories, and sensations by inducing a progressive mindfulness-based detachment (MBD) state in the client. Here the relationship of the individual to the entire content of the mind is changed as opposed to just distressing thoughts. Similar to CBT, TIMBER explicitly aims to change the thought content by systematically using the mindfulness-based graded exposure therapy (MB-GET, [24]). The detached reappraisal of the dysfunctional thoughts and feelings done during the progressive mindfulness-based detachment (MBD) state in the client not only helps to reduce personal identification with depressive/traumatizing ideas and feelings (de-identification) but also gives the individual a wider range of possible viewpoints about himself or herself. The mindfulness-based graded exposure therapy (MB-GET) empowers the individual and reduces the dysfunctions by decreasing the avoidance and arousal responses in the various trigger situations of daily life. Before the client is able to carry out the trauma-specific application of TIMBER, the client is systematically trained in the standardized Yoga and meditation modules in four steps as demonstrated in Fig. 3.2.

3.9 Customization in the TIMBER Therapy

TIMBER interventions are customized based on the client's scores on two scales as well a home practice log specifically designed for this purpose. In this chapter, we mention them briefly, and more detailed description on them can be found in Chap. 4. The two specific scales are *Assessment Scale for Mindfulness Interventions* (ASMI, [8]) and the *Arousal Response during Trauma Memory Reactivation* (ART-MR, [22]). The ASMI is a clinician rated 18-item scale and measures the level of mindfulness including its practice in seven dimensions. Its scores range from 0 to 90: higher the scores, higher is the level of mindfulness. The Arousal Response during Trauma Memory Reactivation (ART-MR) scale is a clinician rated 11-item scale that measures the level of arousal during the controlled reactivation of the traumatic memories using the scripted trauma narrative. The controlled reactivation is done by asking the subject to reflect for 1 min on the *index trauma narrative* (a personalized scripted narrative of the main/index trauma) that was prepared earlier during initial assessment phase using *both the verbal and non-verbal aspects* of the traumatic memories. Then the ensuing arousal responses are allowed to express by the subject for 2–3 min: this step makes the TMs labile and thus prone to change with interventions during the reconsolidation window period which is about 6-h in humans [9]. The ART-MR scores range from 0 to 55; higher scores indicate higher level of arousal. To avoid flooding and re-traumatization in the subjects during the graded exposure to the trauma memories (TMs) while TIMBER therapy is being applied, the arousal responses are kept brief (within 5 min) and scores kept under 30 by using the STOPP module/mini-TIMBER therapy to de-escalate the ensuing arousal responses during the controlled reactivation protocols.

3.10 Achieving the Meditation Skills Before Exposure Therapy Is the Key

After the client is systematically trained in the standardized Yoga and meditation modules in four steps as demonstrated in Fig. 3.1, he/she is encouraged to focus more on the practice of meditation so that they attain the *meditation skill level-3 or higher* and *meditation practice level five or higher* before they are able to apply TIMBER interventions in trauma-specific ways. In StaMP (wellness model) and TIMBER (illness model), emphasis is given on the meditation skills as well as meditation practice because both are complementary to each other and necessary for applying TIMBER effectively. As demonstrated in Fig. 3.3, Pradhan has

Standardized Levels of Mindfulness Skills & Practice (©Basant Pradhan, MD: 2014 onwards) (Pragmatic, evidence based, & studied with *Real-time EEG bio-feedback/rt-EEG-bf*)	
• Able to use **the 'as needed version' of the STOPP module (3 point attention & awareness method with about 10-15 breaths) in at least 4 unpleasant or stressful situations in a week period.**	**Level-10**
• **In a week period, do once daily session of any length at a particular time, for at least 5 times in that week.** For example, if you set a daily practice time for 9pm, you can do it any time in between 8.45pm & 9.15pm	**Level-9**
• **Do a ≥ 5-minute session in the morning, afternoon & evening of the same day**	**Level-8**
• **Do once daily session of any length for 7 consecutive days in a week period.**	**Level-7**
• **Do one session in a week that is at least 20 minute long**	**Level-6**
• **Do once daily session of any length for at least 12 times in a 2-week period. Even a 10 -breath session countsas a practice session**	**Level-5**
• **Able to use the 'as needed version' of the STOPP module (3 point attention & awareness method with about 10-15 breaths) in at least 2 unpleasant or stressful situations in a week period. This is the profound MIDDLE WAY philosophy**	**Level-4**
• **Do once daily session of any length for at least 5 times in a week period . Even a 10 breath session counts. More frequent sessions are better than longer sessions**	**Level-3**
• **Do 8-practice sessions of any length in a two week period (Even a 10 breath session counts: Easiest & most effective way is to end your day with a 20-40 breath session in bed while going to sleep; and begin your day with a 20-40 breath session in bed while going to sleep. No special preparation is necessary.**	**Level-2**
• **Do 4-PRACTICE SESSIONS of any length in a one week period (Even a 10 breath session counts): Easiest way is end your day with a 20-40 breath session in bed while going to sleep; and begin your day with a 20-40 breaths in bed while going to sleep.** • **No special preparation is necessary except making it a routine part of your life**	**Level-1**
Module for Accessing Concentration (MAC Method & STOPP module ©): Customized use of the *Eight-fold Method* of the *Buddha & Patanjali:* **Concentration, Middle Way & Insight Meditation**	
REFERENCES: Books by Pradhan et. al (Springer Publishers). **(1)** ***Yoga and Mindfulness Based Cognitive Therapy (Y-MBCT): A Clinical Guide;*** **(2)** ***Brief Interventions for Psychosis: A Clinical Compendium; (3) Urogenital Pain*** (Chap. 13)	

DATES of Assessment	SKILL LEVELS:1 to 5 (Distraction, Dullness, Detachment, Striving & Middle Way)	PRACTICE LEVELS: 1 to 10	OBSTACLES to Meditation Practice & the ACTION PLAN to Improve Further *(At least Level-3 skills & Level-5 practice needed)*

Fig. 3.3 Standardization of the levels of skills (1-5) and practice (1-10) of meditation

standardized the meditation protocol in terms of five levels of meditation skills and ten levels of meditation practice.

3.11 Trauma-Specific Application of TIMBER Interventions in Three Steps

Once the client has attained the *meditation skill level-3 or higher* and *meditation practice level five or higher*, he/she is encouraged to apply TIMBER interventions in trauma-specific ways using a three-step scheme (as demonstrated in Fig. 3.4).

3.11.1 Structure of the 15 Sessions in TIMBER Therapy

As mentioned before, when it comes to trauma or mindfulness experiences, no two individuals are alike. So the structure described here is just a guide. The number of sessions and what is accomplished in them are very individualistic. For the therapist *the focus should be on the skills built* and not just on how many sessions have been done or how much time has been spent, etc.

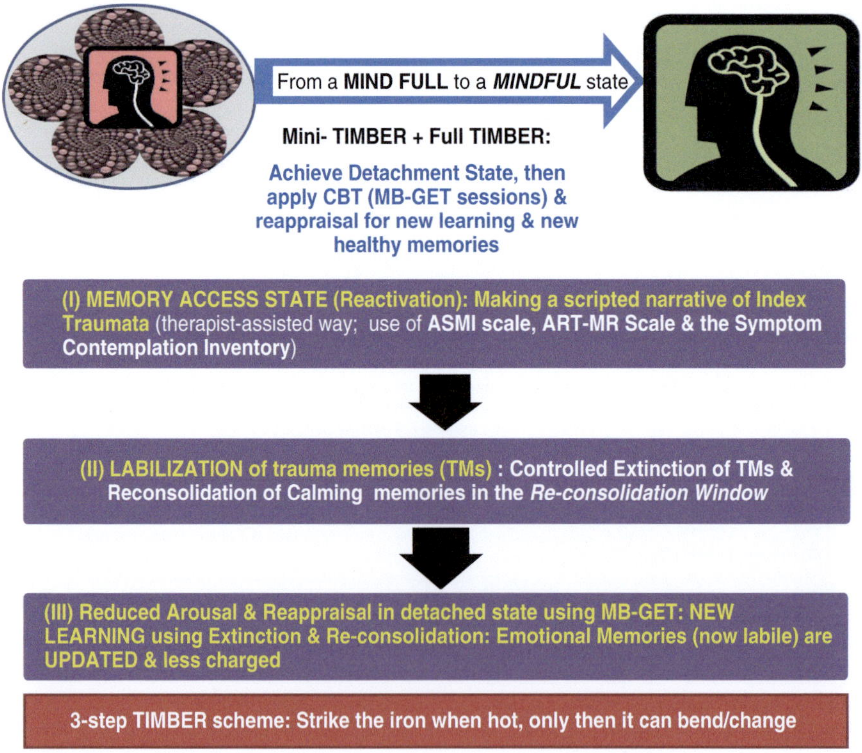

Fig. 3.4 The three-step scheme in applying TIMBER for traumatic memories

Sessions 1–3: The initial sessions of TIMBER aim to achieve three targets—skill building in mindfulness with therapist; working on establishing home practice twice daily (long-practice sessions: once in the morning immediately after waking up and again at night in the bed just before falling asleep, 10 min duration each time), improving sleep, and reducing the stress coming from the physical (somatic) symptoms and anxiety symptoms by daily practice of mindfulness.

Sessions 4–7: To consolidate on skill building and also fine-tune the routine home practice. Then training on the short-practice sessions (3–5 min practice, STOPP module/mini-TIMBER) in the real-life situations as needed to ameliorate the anxiety/anger/sadness/emotional symptoms.

Sessions 8–12: Mindfulness-based graded exposure therapy and restructuring of thoughts by CBT (as part of Full-TIMBER). This is the cornerstone of therapy. In this client and therapist work together to bring up trauma memories in a controlled manner and while in meditative state reframe those memories so that the distress is reduced and self-efficacy in dealing with them is enhanced.

Sessions 13–15: (Total 3-4 booster sessions): The booster sessions are spaced out and determined by client and therapist discussion and decision is made collaboratively. The goals of the booster sessions are to maintain the mindfulness skills during routine practice, to make the as needed practice more skilled and efficient and also to maintain the therapeutic gains and improve the level of functioning.

3.11.2 Data on the Efficacy of TIMBER

As mentioned before, TIMBER was initially designed for treatment of clients with chronic and refractory PTSD in adults and the youth alike. After its efficacy was established in these populations, studies were extended to examine its efficacy in treatment resistant depression and traumatic psychosis. In two recently conducted placebo-controlled randomized controlled trials [14, 22], TIMBER psychotherapy treatment, augmented with medication like a single dose of ketamine infusion at a subanesthetic dose (0.5 mg/kg), has produced significantly longer duration (upto 70 days, mean 33 days) and substantially higher rates (80–85%) of treatment response in chronic PTSD and treatment resistant depression. In this section, we briefly describe the data on the effectiveness of TIMBER for chronic PTSD, treatment resistant depression, and traumatic psychosis: as stand-alone therapy and also in combination with medications like ketamine and with brain stimulation (rTMS) treatments. Most of these data have been published in peer-reviewed journals and cited in the reference section: so we'll not repeat their detailed descriptions here. In this section, we'll provide more description of our analyzed but unpublished data on efficacy of TIMBER which are in the various stages of publication process (Table 3.1).

Combination of TIMBER with rTMS therapy is quite safe and provides extra advantages in terms of not only better efficacy compared to either intervention alone but also it saves therapist's time because it allows for multiple interventions to be done at the same amount of time. In a randomized controlled pilot study done from 2016 to 2018 by our group (Pradhan et al. [25, 26]), in a sample of 14 patients with treatment resistant depression, efficacy of the combined treatment (n = 7) using concurrent

Table 3.1 TIMBER for chronic PTSD, depression, and traumatic psychosis (and chronic addiction)

TIMBER as stand-alone therapy			
Psychiatric condition, study population *References*	Psychiatric condition, study population *References*	Psychiatric condition, study population *References*	Psychiatric condition, study population *References*
Chronic and refractory PTSD, 4 adolescents from age 11–18 years (Case series) [30], *Adolescent Psychiatry* [34]	Chronic and refractory PTSD, 37 patients from age 18–72 years *Unanalyzed and unpublished data*	Chronic treatment resistant depression, 32 patients from 14–74 years [24], *Integrative psychiatry for depression*	Chronic traumatic psychosis, 5 patients from age 16–72 years (Case series) [20]
TIMBER in combination with other interventions			
Ketamine infusion	Psychiatric condition, study population *References*	Psychiatric condition, study population *References*	Psychiatric condition, study population *References*
Ketamine infusion	Chronic and refractory PTSD treatment resistant depression, 20 patients from age 21–60 years (placebo-controlled double blind randomized controlled trial) [14]	Chronic and refractory PTSD, 10 patients from age 21–60 years (placebo-controlled double blind randomized controlled trial) [22]	Biomarker in chronic and refractory PTSD: 47 patients from age 21–60 years (placebo-controlled double blind randomized controlled trial) [25]
Brain stimulation (rTMS)	Chronic treatment resistant depression, 14 patients from age 23–65 years [23, 25, 31, 32]	Chronic and refractory PTSD, 3 patients from age 28–45 years [25]	Chronic addiction, five patients from age 32–55 years (three with opioid addiction and two with nicotine addiction) [25]
Both ketamine and propranolol	Chronic and refractory PTSD, four patients from age 25–48 years [25]		

TIMBER and brain stimulation (rTMS) was compared with rTMS alone ($n = 7$). Compared to the patients receiving only rTMS, the patients in the combined treatment group started improving early (5th session in the combined group vs. 15th session in rTMS only group). Also in the combined group needed less number of rTMS sessions for remission (28.33 ± 2.89 sessions vs. 32.5 ± 3.53 sessions), larger % reduction in the Hamilton Depression Rating Scale (HAM-D17) at completion of 30th treatment session (90.61 ± 3.09 vs. 72.32 ± 20.65, $p = 0.0015$, effect size 3.89, CI = 11.76–24.81), and also longer time to relapse (38 ± 9.90 weeks vs. 10.5 ± 4.95 weeks) ($p = 0.0126$, effect size 3.71, CI = 9.76–45.24). Of note, in the usual standard of care using rTMS only, about 65% patients relapse in 12–20 weeks after completion of the 30th rTMS session, and treatment response is often not apparent until 15th session.

3.11.3 TIMBER Psychotherapy and Biomarkers

In the field of trauma research, improving the clinical diagnostic accuracy through the identification of biomarkers can be helpful for both diagnostic purposes and for evaluating the efficacy of therapeutic modalities. Advancements like these can potentially have a game-changing impact with respect to reliably identifying and treating those at high risk of developing PTSD, traumatic psychosis, or treatment resistant depression (TRD). The clinical improvements seen with TIMBER are associated with a biological change in the brain. In a recent randomized control trial [14, 23], TIMBER psychotherapy alone produced a significant reduction in the 40-min D-Serine plasma concentrations relative to the basal concentrations, which is a further indication that mindfulness meditation produces changes in the basic brain chemistry. In this study, the basal D-serine levels in plasma positively correlated with the pre-treatment severity of PTSD symptoms (Pearson's $r = 0.42$, $p = 0.07$), and patients with basal DSR level ≥3.5 μM displayed not only higher PTSD severity but also shorter duration of response. Basal D-serine levels may serve as a biomarker of the severity of PTSD symptoms and treatment resistant depression as a predictor of clinical response and may represent a significant step toward fulfilling the urgent need to find effective treatments as well as biological markers for PTSD. In the future, investigation of relationship between basal D-serine plasma levels and response to TIMBER therapy should be included in larger inter-institutional studies.

Response to TIMBER has been studied with other biological parameters as well as such multi-system real-time biofeedback measures using the real-time EEG, heart rate variability, and breathing pattern analysis. In the randomized controlled pilot study mentioned earlier (done from 2016 to 2018 by our group (Pradhan et al., [25], unpublished data on 14 patients)), these real-time physiological indices at pre-treatment baseline and at fifth session could predict the treatment response. Of note, in the usual standard of care approach using rTMS only, treatment response is often not apparent until 15th session [27]. Predicting the response early on can empower the treatment provider to make the necessary optimizations to the treatment plan so that treatment outcomes can be improved in these often difficult-to-treat conditions.

TIMBER's application to address the expressions and impact of the traumatic memories in traumatic psychosis and other related conditions is deeply influenced by pathologically ingrained memories. While evidence is building, it is likely that the therapy has a potential to enhance the outcomes for individuals afflicted with other conditions where traumatic memories are the core problem. These can include conditions like borderline personality disorder or drug dependence (as shown in Table 3.1 above), among others. The ongoing clinical and research work by experts in these populations will explore further avenues which have the potential to bridge some of the existing treatment gaps. Of note, these are relatively unexplored areas as far as testing the clinical efficacy of memory-targeted treatment approaches is concerned.

Although the neural circuitry that TIMBER interventions may influence are yet to be probed by functional neuroimaging protocols in the future studies, based on the existing research into the pathways involved in PTSD [28, 29], we postulate that it may involve the fronto-thalamic tri-circuits and the working connections between the amygdala and the prefrontal cortex.

3.12 Conclusions and Future Directions

Drawing from the neurobiologically informed models of trauma memories as well as the existing evidence of efficacy of TIMBER in PTSD, treatment resistant depression, and traumatic psychosis, this chapter has provided information on TIMBER as a stand-alone therapy or in combination with other treatments (such as ketamine infusion, propranolol, and brain stimulation treatment using the TMS). In May 2016, TIMBER was included in the web registry of the California Evidence-Based Clearinghouse for Child Welfare (CEBC, www.cebc4cw.org) [33] as an evidence-based trauma therapy. Some rather difficult-to-treat conditions such as chronic drug dependence and borderline personality disorder more often than not result from severe traumatic experiences as well. As far as testing the clinical efficacy of memory-targeted treatment approaches are concerned, these are relatively unexplored areas and exploring these avenues further has the potential to bridge some of the existing treatment gaps related to these important health conditions. In our ongoing clinical and research work, we have begun to study the feasibility and efficacy of TIMBER in these populations as well and hope to keep our readers informed in future.

References

1. Stein DJ, Ipser JC, Seedat S. Pharmacotherapy for post-traumatic stress disorder (PTSD). Cochrane Database Syst Rev. 2006;(1):CD002795.
2. Strauss C, Rosten C, Hayward M, Lea L, Forrester E, Jones AM. Mindfulness-based exposure and response prevention for obsessive compulsive disorder: study protocol for a pilot randomised controlled trial. Trials. 2015;16:167. https://doi.org/10.1186/s13063-015-0664-7.
3. Brewin CR. Re-experiencing traumatic events in PTSD: new avenues in research on intrusive memories and flashbacks. Eur J Psychotraumatol. 2015;6:27180. https://doi.org/10.3402/ejpt.v6.27180.
4. Chen S, Li L, Xu B, Liu J. Insular cortex involvement in declarative memory deficits in patients with post-traumatic stress disorder. BMC Psychiatry. 2009;9:39.
5. Kenny, Williams. Treatment-resistant depressed patients show a good response to mindfulness-based cognitive therapy. Behav Res Ther. 2007;45(3):617–25.
6. Segal ZV, Williams JM, Teasdale JD. Mindfulness-based cognitive therapy for depression: a new approach to preventing relapse. New York, NY: Guilford Press; 2002.
7. Segal ZV, et al. Cognitive reactivity to sad mood provocation and the prediction of depressive relapse. Arch Gen Psychiatry. 2006;63(7):749–55.
8. Pradhan BK. Yoga and mindfulness based cognitive therapy: a clinical guide. Berlin: Springer; 2014.
9. Monfils MH, Cowansage KK, Klann E, LeDoux JE. Extinction-reconsolidation boundaries: key to persistent attenuation of fear memories. Science. 2009;324:951–5.
10. Schiller D, Cain CK, Curley NG, Schwartz JS, Stern SA, Ledoux JE, Phelps EA. Evidence for recovery of fear following immediate extinction in rats and humans. Learn Mem. 2008;15(6):394–402.

11. Westbrook RF, Iordanova M, McNally G, Richardson R, Harris JA. Reinstatement of fear to an extinguished conditioned stimulus: two roles for context. J Exp Psychol Anim Behav Process. 2002;28:97–110.
12. Hupbach A, Gomez R, Hardt O, Nadel L. Reconsolidation of episodic memories: a subtle reminder triggers integration of new information. Learn Mem. 2007;14:47–53.
13. Kahl KG, Winter L, Schweiger U. The third wave of cognitive behavioural therapies. Curr Opin Psychiatry. 2012;25(6):522–8.
14. Pradhan BK, Mitrev L, Moaddel R, Wainer I. D-Serine is a biomarker for clinical response in (R, S)-ketamine and TIMBER treatment for PTSD and co-morbid depression. Biochim Biophys Acta. 2018a;S1570-9639(18):30035–9.
15. Balasubramaniam M, Telles S, Doraiswamy PM. Yoga on our minds: a systematic review of yoga for neuropsychiatric disorders. Front Psych. 2013;3:117. https://doi.org/10.3389/fpsyt.2012.00117.
16. Brown RP, Gerbarg PL. Sudarshan Kriya Yogic (SKY) breathing in the treatment of stress, anxiety, and depression: clinical applications and guidelines. J Altern Complement Med. 2005;11(4):711–7.
17. Satchidananda S. The Yoga Sutras of Patanjali: translations and commentary. Yogaville, Virginia: Integral Yoga Publications; 1978.
18. Nyanamoli B. The Path of Purification (*Visuddhimagga*). Kandy: Buddhist Publication Society; 1975.
19. Pradhan BK, Sharma A. The time has come for integrating complementary medicine into psychiatry. Adol Psychiat. 2015;5(2):71–2.
20. Pradhan BK, Pinninti NR, Rathod S. Brief interventions for psychosis: a clinical compendium. Switzerland: Springer Publishers; 2016b.
21. McGlynn F, Smitherman T, Gothard K. Comment on the status of systematic desensitization. Behav Modif. 2004;28(2):194–205.
22. Pradhan BK, Wainer IW, Moaddel R, Torjman MC, Goldberg M, Sabia M, Parikh T, Pumariega AJ. Trauma Interventions using Mindfulness Based Extinction and Reconsolidation (TIMBER) psychotherapy prolong the therapeutic effects of single ketamine infusion on post-traumatic stress disorder and comorbid depression: a pilot randomized, placebo-controlled, cross-over clinical trial. Asia Pac J Clin Trials Nerv Syst Dis. 2017;2(3):80–90.
23. Pradhan BK, Makani R, Chatterjee M. Combining mindfulness based cognitive therapy (MBCT) with brain stimulation using concurrent repetitive transcranial magnetic stimulation (rTMS) and focused attention meditation during the rTMS session for refractory depression: a case report. EC Neurology. 2018b;10(4):241–51.
24. Pradhan BK. Depression specific Yoga and mindfulness based cognitive therapy model: Description, data on efficacy and differences from contemporary models (Chapter-24, p. 373-381). In: Greenblatt J, Brogan K, editors. Integrative psychiatry for depression: redefining models for assessment, treatment, and prevention of mood disorders: Taylor & Francis, FL: USA; 2015.
25. Pradhan BK, Biswal B, Elman I, Malik S. (2016): Correlations between the autonomic responses (EEG, heart rate and breath pattern) and treatment response during concurrent mindfulness therapy (TIMBER) and rTMS in resistant depression.
26. Pradhan BK and Malik S (2019). Comparative efficacy of rTMS alone and in combination with EEG-biofeedback guided mindfulness therapy (TIMBER) for resistant depression: A pilot study. Annual conference of the Philadelphia Psychiatric Society.
27. O'Reardon JP, Solvason HB, Janicak PG, et al. Efficacy and safety of transcranial magnetic stimulation in the acute treatment of major depression: a multisite randomized controlled trial. Biol Psychiatry. 2007;62(11):1208–16.
28. Shin LM, Liberzon I. The neurocircuitry of fear, stress and anxiety disorders. Neuropsychopharmacology. 2010;35(2010):169–91.
29. Siegelbaum S, Kandel E. Prefrontal cortex, hippo- campus, and the biology of explicit memory storage. Principles of Neural Science. 5th ed. New York, Chicago, San-Francisco: McGraw-Hill Companies, Inc.; 2013.

30. Pradhan BK, Gray RM, Parikh T, Akkireddi P, Pumariega A. Trauma Interventions using Mindfulness Based Extinction and Reconsolidation (TIMBER) as monotherapy for chronic PTSD in adolescents: A pilot study. Adolescent Psychiat. 2015;5(2):125–31.
31. Pradhan BK, et al. Ketamine, trans-cranial magnetic stimulation (TMS) and depression specific Yoga-mindfulness based cognitive therapy in management of treatment resistant depression: Review and some data on efficacy. Dep Res Treatment. 2015b;2015:842817.
32. Pradhan BK, D'Amico JK, Makani R, Parikh T. Nonconventional interventions for chronic post-traumatic stress disorder (PTSD): Ketamine, repetitive trans-cranial magnetic stimulation (rTMS) and alternative approaches. J Traum Disso. 2015c;17(1):35–54.
33. California Evidence-Based Clearinghouse for Child Welfare2016: Inclusion of TIMBER psychotherapy for PTSD in the program registry website of the California Evidence-Based Clearinghouse for Child Welfare (CEBC, www.cebc4cw.org).
34. Pradhan BK. Clinical considerations for youth with trauma & TIMBER psychotherapy as an emerging evidence-based treatment. In: Blanco RF, Bogacki DF, editors. Prescriptions for children with learning and adjustment problems: a consultant's desk reference. Springfield, Illinois: Charles C. Thomas Publisher; 2017.

Customization and Future Directions in TIMBER

4

4.1 Introduction

Assessment scales in addition to qualitative clinical information are important to help individualize the interventions and evaluate the progress in therapy. However, an assessment scale for trauma that includes only the verbal accounts of client is incomplete and inaccurate and excludes the key processes such as dissociation. Therefore, assessment of trauma should take into account the non-verbal behavior as well because in trauma "The Body Keeps the Score" [1]. Mindfulness-based approaches are gaining relevance for treatment as well as for research purposes in both healthy and clinical populations. The empirical study of mindfulness has rapidly grown, and it is important to have rating scales that are valid and user-friendly. This chapter describes two rating scales: ASMI© (*Assessment Scale for Mindfulness Interventions*, [2]) and ART-MR© (*Arousal Response to Trauma Memory Reactivation*, [3]). Also, it describes a *meditation practice log* that our clients find easy to use. Currently we use these three tools for customizing the TIMBER psychotherapy for our clients. Their names (ASMI and ART-MR) are self-explanatory to an extent. ASMI scale purports to measure dimensionally the level of mindfulness and gives a composite total score as well, whereas the ART-MR scale measures quantitatively the biobehavioral as well as the cognitive-emotional responses, both in the body and mind, during the controlled reactivation of the trauma memories in the therapy sessions. After initial training, the clients can use both scales during their home practice sessions as well using the self-exposure format of TIMBER. The meditation practice log is a self-monitoring tool that helps clients in setting a home practice routine, keeps track of their practice, and eliminates any barriers that they may experience during the practice in order to enhance the quantity as well as quality of their meditation practice. These tools provide rich data from the clients that are used afterward in the session by therapist to tailor the interventions to the unique needs of the clients. In addition to clinical and research use of all three tools (ASMI, ART-MR, and the practice log), we have used ASMI and the home practice log

B. Pradhan et al., *TIMBER Psychotherapy*,
https://doi.org/10.1007/978-3-030-20648-2_4

when we trained staff in the Wellness model of TIMBER (***Sta**ndardized **M**editation **P**ractice*, **StaMP**) and also for our personal practice of meditation in our daily life.

Constructs like personality, mindfulness, trauma experience, personal practice experiences, etc. are often difficult to operationalize and quantify because all of these have significant experiential components. By concretizing these experiences in order to make them measurable in form of a rating scale, one often runs the risk of either missing the items it purports to measure, or the scale may not catch the essence of these experiences. For example, let's hypothesize that a flower on the table is the object of a scientific study. The chief characteristic in this scientific (or objective) approach is to put this object (the flower) to all kinds of analyses, to talk *about* it, to go *around* it, to catch anything *about* it that attracts our intellect and abstract it *away* from the object itself, and, when all is supposedly done, to synthesize these analytically formulated abstractions and take the outcome of the analysis for the object itself. But the question still remains: *Has the complete object* (the flower) *really been caught?* The answer is *no*. These *objective observations* are mere descriptions of the object, in this case the flower, but not the flower itself. So, it may be the case that neither of these three tools (ASMI, ART-MR, or meditation practice log) may be a fully adequate measure of the level of mindfulness or trauma memory reactivation or quality/quantity of meditation practice, all of which are difficult constructs in themselves to be operationalized fully in clinical situations. In particular, neither of them may provide a fully comprehensive assessment of all aspects of the conditions it is purported to measure, and one scale may be particularly indicated in investigations focusing on specific populations such as clinical samples or meditators, etc.

In designing scales that measure human experiences, striking the right balance between the concreteness of measurements and the abstract essence of the experiences these scales purport to measure is never an easy job, rather a Herculean task. However, as each of these tools offers unique advantages and helps us to customize the TIMBER interventions to the needs of our clients, we decided to describe them in this book so that the readers can make an informed decision whether to incorporate them into their own practice. As developer of these three tools, the first author and his colleagues have spent many years querying the patients, healthcare providers, and healthy population as well (who are interested in mindfulness training for improving quality of life) on their needs related to the various aspects these tools purport to measure and testing the prototypes in the real-world settings. Also the second author of the book made some adaptations to the meditation practice log for the needs of his population in a partial hospitalization setting. With respect to these three tools, our description in this chapter will focus mainly on:

(a) The various dimensions these questionnaires cover with respect to mindfulness or trauma
(b) The nature of the relationships between these dimensions
(c) The preliminary data on validity of these measures in our ongoing clinical as well as research work

4.2 Assessment Tools

4.2.1 Assessment Scale for Mindfulness Interventions (ASMI©)

To ensure objectivity and personalization in application of the interventions in the *Yoga and Mindfulness Based Cognitive Therapy* (Y-MBCT, [2]) modules and subsequently in TIMBER, Pradhan in 2012 developed this quantitative scale. Data on the scale was initially published in his monograph, *Yoga and Mindfulness Based Cognitive Therapy* (2014), and subsequently in other work [3–7]. ASMI is an 18-item quantitative, self-rated, and experiential scale that purports to assess the various parameters of meditation, including seven key dimensions of mindfulness for its therapeutic use in health and illness. These dimensions of mindfulness are arrived at based on the existing literature in the *Theravada* as well as the *Mahayana* Buddhism traditions on the various core aspects of mindfulness as a construct [8, 9] and also from the personal experience of mindfulness by the first author who spent a couple of years in a monastery and was planning to become a monk. These *seven dimensions* of mindfulness included in the ASMI are (1) compassion toward self, (2) empathy (compassion toward others), (3) *level of attention*, (4) level of reactivity, (5) mindful observation and interoceptive awareness, (6) awareness and practice of the *Middle Way* (the meditative lifestyle or path of moderation rather than extremes: this is often regarded as the heart of mindfulness practice, [10]), and (7) generalization of one's various learning experiences into the daily life situations. As mentioned in the Chap. 3, the mini-TIMBER or the STOPP module of mindfulness practice is Pradhan's behavioral adaptation of the *Middle Way* philosophy of mindfulness traditions [3]. STOPP is an acronym for *S*tress, *T*hree (or *T*en or *T*wenty) breaths, *O*bserve, *P*ractice, and *P*rogress and specifically helps the clients to quickly de-escalate the arousal symptoms as they arise spontaneously in their daily life situations in response to trauma-related cues/triggers. ASMI scores range from 0 to 90; the higher the scores, the higher is the level of mindfulness. Pradhan and colleagues in their clinical and research work have found that this scale is suitable for use in clients older than 12 years of age (sixth grade reading level or above). Scores can be used not only to assess the levels of mindfulness of the clients in the seven dimensions but also to see their progression during the mindfulness interventions so that specific interventions can be done early during the course of therapy to change these scores for better in the specific dimensions and also to enhance their total scores. Guided by this scale, customizing the Y-MBCT interventions has become possible in terms of treatment planning, deciding upon which one to start with among the seven dimensions and in what sequence to apply them in our clinical work in the various disorders. This has enabled us to move from the "one-size-fits-all" approach to a more "personalized and targeted" clinical approach and also in calculating the appropriate dosing of the therapy. ASMI has been used in clinical subjects as well as normal individuals in multiethnic settings, in different genders and in both adults and youth older than 12 years of age. The actual scale has been illustrated in Fig. 4.1.

Assessment Scale for Mindfulness Interventions (ASMI©, Pradhan, B.K., 2012)

The questions below are about the way you see yourself in the last few days of your life. They're self-rated, self-explanatory & take about 5 minutes to complete. **This form will help personalizing mindfulness tools for you!**

Name: ______________________**; Age:** _____ **Date:**___________ **Education:**________

SCORING

1. Even when things are NOT going the way I want, these days usually I try to be kind and gentle towards myself (0 = Do NOT agree, 1, 2, 3, 4, 5 = Strongly agree)
2. *These days I'm hard on myself about my own flaws or shortcomings (0 = Do NOT agree, 1, 2, 3, 4, 5 = Strongly agree)*
3. These days even when things are NOT going well for me, I'm able to take these as part of life & trying to work through these (0 = Do NOT agree, 1, 2, 3, 4, 5 = Strongly agree)
4. *These days the negative/difficult things about my life often hunt or overwhelm me (0 = Do NOT agree, 1, 2, 3, 4, 5 = Strongly agree)*
5. *These days often I compare myself with others and that makes me feel bad (0 = Do NOT agree, 1, 2, 3, 4, 5 = Strongly agree)*
6. *These days I try too hard for things in my life & I don't give myself any credit for trying (0 = Do NOT agree, 1, 2, 3, 4, 5 = Strongly agree)*
7. Before criticizing somebody, these days I tend to imagine how I would feel if I were in their place (0 = Do NOT agree, 1, 2, 3, 4, 5 = Strongly agree)
8. *These days it is difficult for me to see things from another person's point of view (0 = Do NOT agree, 1, 2, 3, 4, 5 = Strongly agree)*
9. While carrying out tasks in my daily life, these days my level of focus/attention is__ (0= very poor, 1, 2, 3, 4, 5 = excellent)
10. *While carrying out tasks, these days my mind wanders into the past/ future rather than staying in the present moment (0 = Do NOT agree, 1, 2, 3, 4, 5 = Strongly agree)*
11. *These days I'm quite reactive to my life situations around me rather than taking them calmly (0 = Do NOT agree, 1, 2, 3, 4, 5 = Strongly agree)*

Fig. 4.1 The ASMI scale

Assessment Scale for Mindfulness Interventions (ASMI©, Pradhan, B.K., 2012)

SCORING

12. These days I tend to look back and go over the various life situations in a calm & detached manner without getting too reactive or too upset about them
(0 = Do NOT agree, 1, 2, 3, 4, 5 = Strongly agree)
13. These days, I'm quite aware and quick to notice changes in my body and mind when I'm stressed out (for example, my heart or breathing or thoughts becoming faster, my muscles getting tense etc.)
(0 = Do NOT agree, 1, 2, 3, 4, 5 = Strongly agree)
14. *These days my thoughts, feelings and behavior are quite intense and are in the extremes*
(0 = Do NOT agree, 1, 2, 3, 4, 5 = Strongly agree)
15. These days, I'm pretty regular with sleeping, eating and the other habits in my daily life
(0 = Do NOT agree, 1, 2, 3, 4, 5 = Strongly agree)
16. These days, I try to use tools (breathing/ relaxation techniques, coping cards etc.) to help myself with the difficulties coming from my nervous / physical symptoms (0 = Do NOT agree, 1, 2, 3, 4, 5 = Strongly agree)
17. *These days, it is difficult for me to apply to my daily life the helpful things I learn from the various situations*
(0 = Do NOT agree, 1, 2, 3, 4, 5 = Strongly agree)
18. These days, time spent by me daily in practice of meditation, breathing techniques etc. is:
(0 = no practice; 1 = less than 15- minutes; 2 =15-30 minutes; 3 = 31-45 minutes; 4= 46-60 minutes; 5= more than 60 minutes)

How easy was it to fill this form? (0 =not easy at all, 1, 2, 3, 4, 5 =very easy): This item is NOT for scoring.

Comments if any:____________________________________

FOR OFFICE USE ONLY: TOTAL SCORES: _______ /90

Fig. 4.1 (continued)

We recommend that ASMI should be administered at baseline, and after completion of every 5 sessions, until completion of the course of TIMBER therapy (usually 15 sessions including the three booster sessions).

The seven specific dimensions in the ASMI, their scoring, and their relationship to each other are described below:

1. *Compassion toward self* (questions 1 to 6): The higher the scores, the more kind or less critical is the person toward self.
2. *Empathy* (questions 7 and 8): This item reflects compassion toward *others*. The higher the scores, the higher is the empathy. We often notice that clients afflicted with trauma have high level of empathy (compassion toward others) but low level of self-compassion.

3. *Level of attention* (questions 9 and 10): The higher the scores on this, the higher is the level of attention, and the less is the mind wandering.
4. *Level of reactivity* (question 11): The higher the scores on this, the higher is the level of reactivity or arousal, and the lower is the level of responsiveness.
5. *Mindful observation* (question 12) and *interoceptive awareness* (question 13): These two items in this very important dimension of mindfulness reflect the client's ability to *just calmly note things in mind* (such as thoughts, feelings) and body (such as bodily sensations) rather than reacting to them in repetitive and emotional ways or ruminating over them. These two items often go together. The higher the scores on questions 12 and 13, the higher is the level of calmness, neutral observation, and responsiveness, and the lower is the level of reactivity and arousal.
6. Awareness and practice of the *Middle Way* (questions 14 and 15): The higher the scores on this, the higher is the level of mindfulness practice with respect to regularity and quality, the less is the level striving during meditation practice, and the higher is the rhythmicity of the client's daily life activities such as sleeping, eating, etc.
7. *The level of generalization* of one's various learning experiences (questions 16 to 18): The higher the scores in these items, the higher is the extent of generalization of the therapeutic gains into client's daily life situations.

Thus, ASMI generates a quantitative score that range from 0 to 90, and the higher are the scores, the higher is the level of mindfulness in the individual. Among the 18 questions, *half of them* (nine questions 2, 4, 5, 6, 8, 10, 11, 14, and 17; these items are in *italics*) *are scored in reverse manner*. In these nine items, if person marks "0," that is taken as "5" and vice versa.

4.2.2 The Arousal Response to Trauma Memory Reactivation (ART-MR©) Scale

To keep the hyperarousal symptoms low and controlled during the trauma memory reactivation protocol of TIMBER, in 2013 Pradhan with consultation from a trauma therapist Richard Gray, PhD, developed this quantitative scale. Data on this scale was initially published in 2015 [11] and subsequently in other works [3, 4, 12]. The ART-MR scale is a clinician-rated scale that measures the level of biobehavioral and cognitive-emotional arousal responses dimensionally and also generates a total score from its 11 items during the controlled reactivation of the traumatic memories using a scripted narrative of the index trauma. This scripted narrative is prepared in a personalized way for each client during the initial assessment phase using both the verbal and non-verbal aspects of traumatic memories. The controlled reactivation is done by asking the subject to reflect for 1 min on this scripted narrative. Then the ensuing arousal responses are allowed to express by the subject for 2–3 min: this step makes the TMs labile and thus prone to change with interventions during the reconsolidation window period which is about 6-hours in humans [13]. Its scores range from 0 to 55; higher scores indicate higher level of arousal. The actual scale has been illustrated in Fig. 4.2.

ART-MR scale takes into account the verbal as well as non-verbal behavior in response to the controlled reactivation of the trauma memories in treatment settings. This is a unique feature of ART-MR as it is the only scale we are aware of

Arousal Response during Trauma Memory Reactivation© (ART-MR, Pradhan and Gray, 2013) 1

Clients's Name:____________________;Gender:________; Level of Education:__________; Date:____________

Instructions : *ART-MR scale requires the rater to carefully observe the client during the controlled reactivation process of trauma memories in the reconsolidation window. This scale has 11 items, takes about 5-minutes to complete* and the *scores range from 0 to 55*: higher the scores, higher is the level of arousal. While administering this scale, the arousal parameters to observe in the client involve *verbal as well as non-verbal, verbal, emotional and physiological changes in the client after 1-minute exposure to* ***a brief narrative of the index trauma***. ART-MR was specifically designed to prevent excessive arousal and re-traumatization during trauma therapy. Dr. Pradhan's **STOPP module (mini-TIMBER) of *TIMBER*© therapy** helps bring back the calmness within a few minutes during this controlled arousal.

Please indicate if the following three items are present: (a) Client has one or a few *specific* memories about an index trauma (involving severe abuse, death or immanent destruction). True ☐ False ☐

(b) The trauma is the source of nightmares and flashbacks in which client *re-lives* the trauma or shows aspects of arousal (even if client doesn't fully recall it). True ☐ False ☐

(c) *Specific* and predominant cues (perceptual/ *situational*) of *Index Trauma* that caused arousal response most recently and can be used for controlled *for trauma memory reactivation*: ______________________________

(d) Any Meds/Other factors that can interfere with responses to ART-MR questions

During your observation, please rate the following factors *by documenting the changes on the 11 parameters listed below*. For all the changes observed, whenever possible, please note the details of the changes & their sequence, if any. **On a scale of 0 (means 'none') to 5 (means 'very much without question'), please rate the following items:**

1. **Eye response** (change in size, movements, open/closed, change in eye contact, downcast):

   None Little Very much
   0--------------1----------------2---------------3---------------4----------------5

2. **Eye brows response** (e.g. furrowed, frowned, raised, lowered etc.):

   None Little Very much
   0--------------1----------------2---------------3---------------4----------------5

3. **Pupillary change during arousal** (widened, contracted, etc.): **from baseline size___mm to ___mm**

   None Little Very much
   0--------------1----------------2---------------3---------------4----------------5

4. **Facial muscle tone** (e.g. tightened, relaxed, clenched, etc.):

   None Little Very much
   0--------------1----------------2---------------3---------------4----------------5

5. **Facial color change** (if applicable: reddened, paled, purple, etc.).

   None Little Very much
   0--------------1----------------2---------------3---------------4----------------5

6. **Movement response in the various body parts** (e.g. fidgeting fingers, shaking feet/legs, shrugging shoulders, clenching teeth, biting lips, biting tongue, biting nails, body rigidity)

   None Little Very much
   0--------------1----------------2---------------3---------------4----------------5

7. **Change in posture** (erect, leaning left, leaning right, slouching, leaning back, leaning forward)

   None Little Very much
   0--------------1----------------2---------------3---------------4----------------5
   Sequence of change, if any____

Fig. 4.2 The ART-MR scale

Arousal Response during Trauma Memory Reactivation© (ART-MR, Pradhan and Gray, 2013) 2

8. **Change of breathing** (rate increased, rate decreased; any change of breathing location— e.g. high chest, middle chest, belly, etc.)

None Little Very much
0--------------1----------------2---------------3---------------4----------------5

9. **Change in heart rate (HR) during 1-minute exposure: Please see the table below for documentation**

0 (No change); 1(HR changed by 1-5 from baseline); **2** (HR changed by 6-10 from baseline); **3** (HR changed by 11-15 from base line); **4** (HR changed by 16-20 from base line); **5** (HR changed by > 20 from base line)

10. **Perspiration (sweaty hands etc.)**

None Little Very much
0--------------1----------------2---------------3---------------4----------------5

11. **Predominant emotion(s) during assessment (anger, fear, hatred, sadness, surprise** etc.)

Strong and involuntary (reflex-like) emotional response either spontaneously with very mild trigger (e.g. eyes welling up with tears or outright crying, changes in breathing, facial color, changes in the pace and tone of voice, a need to stop the exposure because of intense arousal, shaking, sweating, acting as if client is seeing or hearing the events all over again).

None Little Very much
0--------------1----------------2---------------3---------------4----------------5

Sequence of change, if any:____

____

TOTAL SCORES (from 11 questions) with 1-minute exposure = ☐ / **55**

Documentation on changes in Heart Rate (HR):

	Baseline (Pre-exposure)	During Controlled Exposure (1-minute exposure / cycle)		5-minutes Post-exposure	
HEART RATE (per minute)	**Cycle#1**	Highest HR ☐	**Mean Rise** ☐	Highest HR ☐	**Mean Rise** ☐
	Cycle#2	Highest HR ☐	**Mean Rise** ☐	Highest HR ☐	**Mean Rise** ☐
	Cycle#3	Highest HR ☐	**Mean Rise** ☐	Highest HR ☐	**Mean Rise** ☐

SPECIAL NOTES:

- **Three Steps in One Mini-TIMBER cycle: Step:1:** Number of standardized breaths needed to establish calmness while stopping bodily movements & using five neutral words (______); **Step-2:** 1-minute of controlled exposure using scripted trauma narrative, and
  Step-3: Number of standardized breaths needed to re-establish calmness while stopping bodily movements and using five neutral words for reappraisal of trauma memories (_____)
- Time taken to control the hyper-arousals and bring back to baseline: ____minute(s)
- Number of mini-TIMBER cycles done during a re-activation session (5 mins/cycle): (____)
- Any additional **Physical or Non-Verbal** symptoms during the TIMBER session: (__________)

Difficulties doing the mini-TIMBER, if any:____

Fig. 4.2 (continued)

that covers both the verbal and non-verbal activation from trauma memories in a comprehensive manner. The other unique feature of ART-MR scale is that it plays a vital role in avoiding the overflooding and re-traumatization of the client in treatment settings. Re-traumatization in treatment settings is common in other therapies like the prolonged exposure therapy which not only causes treatment-emergent worsening of PTSD but also comes in the way of engaging the clients effectively into the therapeutic process. To avoid overflooding and re-traumatization in the subjects during the graded exposure to the trauma memories (TMs), while TIMBER therapy is being applied, the arousal responses are kept brief (within 5 min) and scores kept under 30 by using the STOPP module/mini-TIMBER therapy to de-escalate the ensuing arousal responses during the controlled reactivation protocols. Of note, the STOPP module of mindfulness is Pradhan's behavioral adaptation of the Middle Way philosophy of mindfulness traditions, which he has successfully applied in clinical situations within the age range of 6–80 years [3]. As described in detail in Chap. 3, controlled reactivation of the trauma memories makes these long-term memories of trauma *labile* and thus more amenable to change by using a balanced combination of extinction and reconsolidation methods of TIMBER.

4.3 Meditation Home Practice Log

For ensuring further objectivity in application and generalization of the Y-MBCT interventions, Pradhan developed this standardized meditation practice log in 2012 which since then is being used by him and colleagues in their ongoing clinical and research work. This practice log is self-explanatory and easy to use. In this practice log (Fig. 4.3), emphasis is placed on mainly two aspects: how to ensure a daily practice meditation in a user-friendly way and how to remove the obstacles to meditation in a systematic and personalized manner based on the client's mindfulness profile and the many personality and psychosocial factors.

In addition to other data from our ongoing research, data from use of this practice log since 2009 includes over 500 patients and over 300 healthy subjects. This has provided us with evidence that 5–10 min of daily practice of meditation over 4–6 weeks can be effective in educational settings (high school or medical students, etc.) as well as some clinical settings (especially in generalized anxiety disorder and mild/moderate level of depression). However, 10–15 min practice daily over 6–8 weeks is an optimal duration to elicit long-lasting psychological benefits. Longer sessions such as 25–30 min per day for at least 4–6 weeks may be especially useful in more serious clinical settings (such as PTSD, severe depression, severe OCD etc.), particularly because those evoke positive functional and structural brain changes (neuroplasticity) [14].

MINDFULNESS: Standardized Practice Schedule (©BasantPradhan,M.D.,2012onwards)

Please fill this **weekly home practice log** for your whole day practice when you get a chance. It is a good way to practice daily in bed for the ***routine practice*** without any special preparation (**60-70 breaths**, lying down posture, just **feel physically the breath sensations** as you breathe from belly slowly with mouth closed). You can practice as many times you can for the ***as needed practice*** **(10-15 breaths, with mouth closed)**. Please make a note of *any distractions* (which can be any of the **five things**: *thoughts, feelings, sensations, urges to do things and memories*) that comes up between you & your breath during practice. Please maintain this practice log **for at least the first 4-weeks of practice.** Please do this until your practice has become regular for at least 4-6 weeks.

Name:______________________ **Practice week: from date** ____________ **to date**____________

Day/Date/Total duration of Meditation Practice	**Daily Frequency of Meditation Practice**	**COMMENTS (difficulties/distractions encountered** during your practice at home / while doing the tasks of daily life)
Friday Total duration of practice:______minutes	Practiced____ times today Used in daily life: No Yes	
Saturday Total duration of practice:______minutes	Practiced____ times today Used in daily life: No Yes	
Sunday Total duration of practice:______minutes	Practiced____ times today Used in daily life: No Yes	
Monday Total duration of practice:______minutes	Practiced____ times today Used in daily life: No Yes	
Tuesday Total duration of practice:______minutes	Practiced____ times today Used in daily life: No Yes	
Wednesday Total duration of practice:______minutes	Practiced____ times today Used in daily life: No Yes	
Thursday Total duration of practice:______minutes	Practiced____ times today Used in daily life: No Yes	

Total duration of practice for the above WEEK: ___________ minutes

Current target situations for as needed practice: ____

The single biggest obstacle to your mindfulness practice is/will be ____________________________

Happy Practicing Mindfulness! Pradhan-Basant@Cooperhealth.edu

Fig. 4.3 Meditation home practice log

4.4 Three Aspects of the TIMBER Psychotherapy

TIMBER psychotherapy comprises of the Wellness model (StaMP) and the disorder-specific Y-MBCT model (TIMBER proper) and has three dimensions:

1. The theoretical and philosophical aspects
2. The techniques
3. The practice aspects

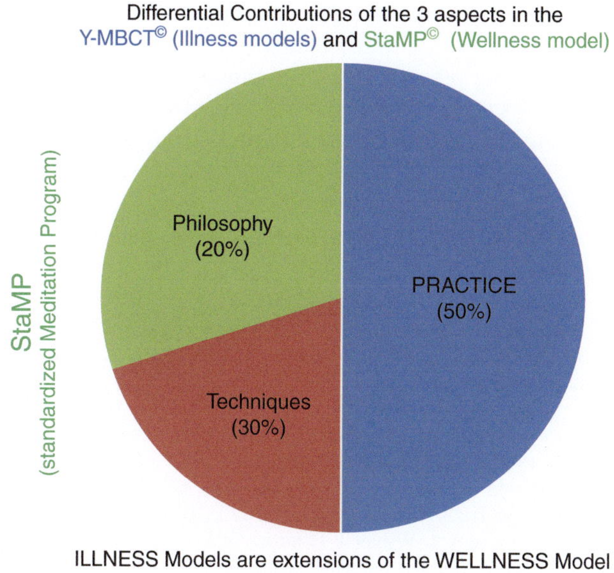

Fig. 4.4 Three aspects of the TIMBER psychotherapy

In our experience, the differential contributions of the theoretical and philosophical underpinnings that client has to understand are about 20%, those of the techniques they have to learn are about 30%, and those of the practice they have to master are about 50%. The relative importance of these dimensions is illustrated in Fig. 4.4.

4.5 Conclusions and Future Directions

Standardized rating scales for mindfulness-based or trauma-related work are needed to evaluate the efficacy of the various interventions and also for cross-study comparisons. It is challenging to find the right balance in concretizing human experience such as mindful state and not losing the essence of the experience. The two scales (ASMI and ART-MR) and the meditation practice log described in this chapter have clinical evidence supporting their use but have limitations in that their psychometric properties have not been established yet. Clinicians can use these scales for now, while the authors continue to strive to build the empirical evidence for these scales. Also, we have started our work on delivering TIMBER psychotherapy via video conferencing for clients located in remote areas [15] as well as studying the therapeutic responses to TIMBER with a greater number of biological markers.

Our future work on these instruments and on TIMBER will focus on the following aspects:

- To study in more detail the psychometric properties of ASMI and ART-MR scales
- To work more on training other healthcare professionals on TIMBER and on biological markers of its response so that it will allow for more generalization as well as prognostication and preemptive treatment planning, respectively

References

1. Van der Kolk B. The body keeps the score. New York: Viking Penguin; 2014.
2. Pradhan BK. Yoga and mindfulness based cognitive therapy: a clinical guide. Switzerland: Springer Publishers; 2014.
3. Pradhan BK, Wainer IW, Moaddel R, Torjman MC, Goldberg M, Sabia M, Parikh T, Pumariega AJ. Trauma Interventions using Mindfulness Based Extinction and Reconsolidation (TIMBER) psychotherapy prolong the therapeutic effects of single ketamine infusion on post-traumatic stress disorder and comorbid depression: a pilot randomized, placebo-controlled, cross-over clinical trial. Asia Pac J Clin Trials Nerv Syst Dis. 2017;2(3):80–90.
4. Pradhan BK, Mitrev L, Moaddel R, Wainer I. D-Serine is a biomarker for clinical response in (R, S)-ketamine treatment of post-traumatic stress disorder and co-morbid depression. Biochim Biophys Acta. 2018;S1570-9639(18):30035–9.
5. Pradhan BK. Depression specific Yoga and mindfulness based cognitive therapy model: description, data on efficacy and differences from contemporary models (Chapter 24). In: Greenblatt J, Brogan K, editors. Integrative psychiatry for depression: redefining models for assessment, treatment, and prevention of mood disorders. FL: Taylor & Francis; 2015. p. 373–81.
6. Pradhan BK, Sharma A. The time has come for integrating complementary medicine into psychiatry. Adolesc Psychiatry (Editorial). 2015;5(2):71–2.
7. Pradhan BK, et al. Ketamine, trans-cranial magnetic stimulation (TMS) and mindfulness based cognitive therapy in management of treatment resistant depression: review and some data on efficacy Dep Res Treat. 2015;1–14. Epub 2015 Oct 5.
8. Analayo B. Satipatthana: the direct path to realization. Birmingham, UK: Windhorse publications; 2003.
9. Thera U. The path of freedom (Vimuttimagga). Kandy, Sri Lanka: Budhist Publication Society; 1961.
10. Lama D. The middle way: faith grounded in reason (trans: Jinpa T). Boston: Wisdom Publications; 2009.
11. Pradhan BK, Gray RM, Parikh T, Akkireddi P, Pumariega A. Trauma Interventions using Mindfulness Based Extinction and Reconsolidation (TIMBER) as monotherapy for chronic PTSD in adolescents: a pilot study. Adolescent Psychiat. 2015;5(2):125–31.
12. Pradhan, B.K. (2016): TIMBER (Trauma Interventions Using Mindfulness Based Extinction/Re-consolidation of trauma memories) therapy for chronic and refractory PTSD was included in the program registry website of the California Evidence-Based Clearinghouse for Child Welfare (CEBC, www.cebc4cw.org).
13. Monfils MH, Cowansage KK, Klann E, LeDoux JE. Extinction-reconsolidation boundaries: key to persistent attenuation of fear memories. Science. 2009;324:951–5.
14. Tang YY, Ma YH, Wang J, Fan YX, Feng SG, Lu QL. Short-term meditation training improves attention and self-regulation. Proc Natl Acad Sci U S A. 2007;104:17152–6.
15. Kunaparaju, S., Pradhan, B.K., Parikh, S. (2017): Using video-conferencing to deliver TIMBER psychotherapy for PTSD: A Case Report on an Indian Client. Proceedings of the Annual Meeting of the American Psychiatric Association, San Diego.

Discussion and Illustrations of the Therapeutic Processes in TIMBER

5

5.1 Nosological and Diagnostic Problems in Trauma Care

Chapter 1 clearly delineated the different types of trauma and its varied effects. A book on trauma is never complete without discussion of complex trauma or complex PTSD [1], probably one of the most devastating sufferings of the human mind that has a wide array of health consequences, both mental and physical. Complex trauma results from the exposure to multiple and severe traumatic events during the childhood which are often of an invasive and interpersonal nature. These traumatic events such as severe abuse or profound neglect are pervasive and often occur by a caregiver, thus interfering with the child's ability to form a secure attachment [2]. Complex trauma can disrupt many critical aspects of the child's development including both physical and mental growth. The physical health adversities include severe conditions such as failure to thrive, stunted growth, childhood-onset metabolic syndrome, etc. On the other hand, the problems of mental development can be severe problems in affect regulation and the formation of a sense of self and personality. The results are a variety of psychiatric conditions such as PTSD, recurrent or resistant depression, chronic drug addiction, borderline personality disorder, and traumatic psychosis [3–5]. Complex trauma victims often are too young, too shocked, and too demoralized. They are often too focused on simply surviving, and they are in a constant state of threat with responses of fight, flight, or freeze to the benign and routine stressors of life. Their thoughts and behavior are typically reflective of their excessive safety behaviors or their preoccupation to know or recall what they were feeling at the time of the traumatic exposure: *truly they are the captives of their pathologically ingrained trauma memories which dictate their lives.*

The issue of diagnosis of trauma, especially complex trauma, and the plethora of health conditions ensuing from it have been contentious over more than a century. For example, back in the twentieth century, many (if not all) of the female clients who reported trauma histories and exhibited complex trauma symptoms were labeled as *hysterics* and *borderline personality disorders*. Although borderline personality disorder results from trauma and can often coexist with PTSD, correctly

B. Pradhan et al., *TIMBER Psychotherapy*,
https://doi.org/10.1007/978-3-030-20648-2_5

diagnosing the individuals is critically important, especially for their appropriate management. For example, diagnosing complex PTSD as a personality disorder not only can be demoralizing for the client ("My core self is defective") but also may misdirect the therapist by making the personality the main focus rather than the trauma-related adaptations that affect but are distinct from the core self.

Ironically, the current psychiatric classification systems such as DSM and ICD don't include complex PTSD yet as a formal diagnosis. Both these classificatory systems are categorical in nature, while the different conditions that develop from the underlying trauma are best conceptualized on a continuum or dimensional perspective.

When it comes to trauma, no two individuals are exactly alike with their symptoms. The interactions between trauma, developmental phases of life, and existing support systems available to the individual to deal with trauma are complex. These interactions can lead to a variety of outcomes for the individual exposed to trauma. The mediating factors from trauma to eventual psychopathology such as PTSD or complex PTSD, generalized anxiety, major depressive disorder, bipolar disorder, etc. need to be further delineated to better allow us to fine-tune the therapeutic interventions for the various stages of development and maintaining of the psychopathologies. When therapist views trauma on a dimensional perspective, the core elements of trauma experience are addressed, and individual differences in symptoms become less important to focus on core pathology.

5.2 Some Problems with the Current System of Care

Healthcare systems in many countries like the United States and United Kingdom have undergone significant changes in the last decade, and use of electronic health records is one such example. Computerized electronic health records are a transformative technology with significant benefits including clarity, standardization, accountability, and ease of use both for collaborative clinical care and for research purposes. However, they have major disadvantages as well, mainly by creating a system of care that is more technical than human or relational. For example, the healthcare professionals spend far more time in front of their computer screens for the purpose of completing the documentation and checking all the boxes that the system requires them to check and this interferes in their ability to form and maintain therapeutic (healing) relationship with clients and their families. A healing relationship is essential to provide safe emotional space for the individual to deal with the impact of trauma and build resilience. Therapeutic relationship is typically conducive to healing if it is established and maintained with the specific providers over a period of time. However, the current healthcare experience of clients or patients in many countries such as the United States is very fragmented and lacks continuity [6]. It can feel like clients are on an assembly line. Let us take the example of a patient who goes to emergency department (ED) for suicidal ideation in depression and is referred to a community agency for outpatient level of care. This client sees an intake coordinator for intake and referred to intensive outpatient therapy (IOP).

In the IOP setting, the client sees a therapist for about 12 weeks and a psychiatrist for medication monitoring and at the end is referred to an outpatient program where he/she can start with a new therapist and psychiatrist. In a 4-month period that started with a crisis visit, the client is with his/her third psychiatrist, second therapist, and third intake coordinator! Where does this system allow for a healing relationship to develop and strengthen over time? In this fragmented system, the clients often do not have a say in choosing their mental healthcare provider(s) and have to follow the process laid out for them. We need to be very aware of these complexities, the fragmentation of the system, and take active steps to mitigate against the negative effects of these. These issues with the system that come in the way of effective care delivery, especially in trauma care, can be summarized as:

(a) Focus being on documentation and not on the relationship building
(b) Fragmented care ("split treatment")
(c) Lack of continuity

Secure relationship with adults during formative years leads to secure attachment, and thereby it is the foundation for healing relationship with therapist. Healing requires relationships—relationships which lead to trust, hope, and a sense of being known or understood. However, adverse childhood experiences such as abuse and neglect disrupt this foundation resulting the client's inability to trust the nurturing figures including the therapists. Individuals dealing with sequelae of trauma often describe their mental health system experience as traumatizing [7] and contribute to the *tertiary level* trauma. Viewing healthcare as an evolving whole instead of only as fragmented parts can help us to feel hope where now there is cynicism. Understanding the fundamental problem of fragmentation in our healthcare system is an important first step for re-establishing a better and trauma informed healthcare.

5.3 Some Proposed Solutions to These Problems

The following steps are important in addressing some of the current deficiencies in the system. Probably the first and foremost task is to establish trust in the therapeutic relationship because that has been already lost long back in almost all clients with severe trauma due to lack of secure attachments in formative years. Next important step can be for the therapist to acknowledge these problems in the existing system. This way the therapist is validating client's healthcare experience. For many individuals with trauma who had their experiences invalidated, this is a corrective experience that helps them to build trust with therapist, who represents an authority or nurturing figure. After these first two crucial steps have been taken care of, the next step is to ensure that everything is done to maintain the continuity of care, while the client is with the service. In several instances the client may be in the same organization but going to a different program, and in those instances a warm and empathic handoff where the client is introduced to the next therapist while still being in the program and discussing the progress of therapy especially what helped and what didn't help in the healing process can go to some extent in mitigating the effects of a fragmented system of care. There are some innovative pilot programs that are being evaluated to address the current deficiencies in the system and create an integrated care system that addresses the four major groups of client needs: mental health needs, addiction service needs, physical health needs, and social service needs. There is a federal innovative program in the United States called the CCBHC (Certified Community Behavioral Health Center) that addresses all these needs and is described in Chap. 7 in more detail. In the United Kingdom, many places are establishing a Single Point of Access (SPOA) to address the same issue. SPOA [8] in the United Kingdom is like a "one-stop shop" and provides timely access to intensive community-based care management, assertive community treatment (ACT), and/or housing services and supports for adults with severe mental illness. Another important task is to make the therapeutic experience between the client and the clinician the main focus (rather than making the documentation tasks the main focus). Trauma therapies need to be targeted, time limited, and relational as well. Given the limitations of our current system of care and limited time that the therapist gets with client, it is important for therapist to work in a "triage/priority-based paradigm" while still maintaining the core therapeutic relationship so that the core symptoms are more effectively addressed in the least amount of time.

5.4 How TIMBER Differs from the Contemporary Trauma Therapies?

Although CBT is the most evidence based among all psychotherapies, unfortunately, because of too much emphasis on achieving the treatment goals, the use of relational principles and techniques is not yet common in the cognitive-behavioral trauma therapy, nor are the therapist attunement and empathy always highly valued. Similarly, although psychodynamic therapists do have a relational focus, more often than not, they are not goal driven and don't consider therapy titration (dosing) or staging important.

One of the criticisms leveled against psychotherapy today, particularly CBT, is for the process being too technical with less emphasis on the experience which in turn may reduce the patient engagement into the therapeutic process, more so in trauma therapy.

Taking these issues into considerations, the psychotherapeutic processes in TIMBER try to strike a balance with respect to these important limitations in the existing trauma therapy.

TIMBER is *translational, targeted, and time limited* (**3 Ts of TIMBER**) *but relational as well.* TIMBER is translational because it incorporates the basic sciences and neurobiological research into its methodology. It combines Yoga and mindfulness with the pragmatism of CBT, and in our field there is a dearth of therapies whose efficacies have been tested with biological marker(s). In the spirit of applying personalized medicine, TIMBER is primarily experiential and customized or tailored to the client's individual experiences in the here and now. The client experience is the clinical information that is used by the therapist to determine and drive the therapeutic interventions. Many of the unique features of TIMBER have been elaborated in Chaps. 3 and 4. In TIMBER therapy, the therapist helps the trauma-afflicted individual feel safe and secure in the very first session and thereby establish deeper and more empathic connections. TIMBER requires the therapist's own practice of meditation using the Standardized Meditation Program (StaMP) which enables the therapist to access mindful state in their own minds and also enhances the therapist's ability to teach these specific techniques in first session. This also facilitates the empathic connection or therapeutic alliance, and the insession practice with the client mitigates their learned hopelessness, anger, and frustration as well.

The points mentioned above are quite important in order to learn and practice TIMBER in its true sense. This kind of approach allows the therapist to bring to the therapy session a meditative state of mind (*alert but relaxed and nonreactive*) which is more responsive than reactive. In the therapy session, client and therapist are mutually impacted by their respective mind states. Traumatized individuals have high level activity of amygdala (threat detection system in brain) and are more reactive to stimuli that are perceived as threatening [9]. A meditative mind-set of the therapist helps to lower the activity of the amygdala for the client and augment the prefrontal cortical activity [10]. Lowered amygdalar activity is perceived by the client as a state of relative neutrality and psychological safety. An overactive amygdala leads to a hyperarousal state with sealing over of trauma memories and forces the individual to function in a survival mode by use of the fright, fight, or flight responses even in benign situations of daily life. With lowered amygdalar activity (lowered reactivity) and enhanced prefrontal activity (enhanced attention and open awareness) brought forward by the meditative contemplation, the client becomes progressively open to further explore, access, and express in relatively less emotionally intense ways the long-suppressed trauma details. This provides the therapist and client with a rich and personalized database to work through during the therapeutic work to promote healing. This is the stage where the therapist would teach the client the techniques (nuts and bolts) to be mindful as described in detail below. Learning the techniques gives the ability to the client to (a) practice the technique at home and become self-efficacious in using it and (b) the ability to deal with the trauma-associated experiences in a detached manner. The result is decrease in avoidance and safety behaviors, sense of control, and empowerment, and it enhances their sense of hope.

5.5 A Case-Based Illustration of TIMBER

The case of *Cathy* (for confidentiality reasons, actual name is not being mentioned here)**:** this particular case illustrates the incorporation of TIMBER psychotherapy into a routine medication management clinic in an intensive outpatient program. The client was able to learn and benefit from TIMBER therapy provided by second author, while she was seeing a regular therapist as part of the program. The second author worked with the therapist to enhance his understanding of the therapy and prevent cross-communication between two therapists. The client was able to show resolution of her symptoms, reduce medication significantly, and improve overall quality of her life through TIMBER.

A 46-year-old Caucasian female living with her husband and two teenaged children, son aged 19 and daughter aged 17 presented with anxiety and constant sense of dread, triggered panic attacks, intrusive memories of childhood trauma, depressed mood, insomnia, worthlessness, and inappropriate guilt. Diagnoses at admission were severe PTSD, major depressive disorder, and generalized anxiety. PTSD symptoms were being the most distressing and disabling. She described her condition as being a prisoner of her own mind as depicted in the painting she drew of herself (Fig. 5.1).

Cathy had several triggers for flashbacks including visit to doctor's offices and the prospect of vital signs being taken. Her enduring trauma was childhood sexual abuse by father from age 4 and lasted several years. Her mother described as functional alcoholic with sociopathic tendencies, and she reportedly used her daughter for medical experimentation. In addition, the client used to be locked up in her room for several days at a time as punishment. Before she came to services, she was followed up by a psychiatrist in private practice who prescribed daily doses of vortioxetine 20 mg, aripiprazole 5 mg, and clonazepam 3 mg. According to the client, her psychiatrist did not want to lower her medication, and hence she

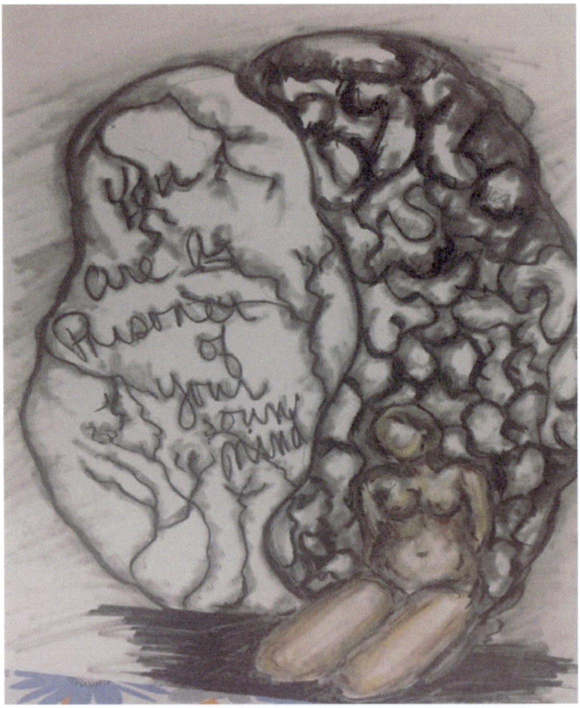

Fig. 5.1 This "self-portrait" reflects her perception about herself before she started TIMBER therapy

reluctantly went along with his recommendation. However she reported significant lethargy that impaired the quality of her life. She was admitted to the intensive outpatient program that included seeing a therapist weekly and attending one or two groups per week. The second author did psychiatric evaluation and medication monitoring and provided TIMBER as part of these visits. In the 4 months, she was in the program, and she had a total of five visits with the TIMBER therapist who kept in regular touch with the individual therapist to inform about the work done in the sessions. The individual therapist reinforced the practice of the technique to help the client address trauma and complemented this through CBT interventions to address other psychosocial issues such as her son disclosing that he was bisexual. The client was in the program for a total of 4 months during which time she developed strong mindfulness skills and was to come off the clonazepam and aripiprazole completely and stayed on only on antidepressant Vortioxetine.

At the time of her discharge, she reported that PTSD and depressive symptoms resolved almost completely. Her functioning in realm of work and interpersonal functioning improved significantly. She reported feeling liberated psychologically and started engaging in her hobby of painting. She said "I was faceless, nameless and voiceless when I came to the program as picture (Fig. 5.1) shows. Now I am a different person. I know exactly what I want and I am going for it in life. I am so much more happy and it was wonderful getting this therapy." Also for the first time in her life, she started working on pursuing a career in medical illustration. From therapist's point of view, she had symptom resolution and improved functioning and was more resilient to deal with life problems. This particular case illustrates that TIMBER can be provided in concert with other individual or group therapies by working with other therapists and this way it can be incorporated into regular med monitoring visits without adding significant time burden or disruption.

5.6 Conclusion

Psychotherapeutic process at its core rests on developing a deep emotional connection between a therapist and the client. This connection helps the client work through the effects of trauma and should be long enough for the client to benefit from therapy. The current system of care places some barriers in providing this type of relationship and for required length of time. In this chapter we have provided a brief overview of the existing lacunae in current system of care and provided clinical illustration as well as some recommendations to provide a bird's-eye view on utility of TIMBER in the real-world situations. We do recognize that TIMBER still has many miles to go in its future path in order to generalize its effects and efficacy.

In the next chapter, we discuss how TIMBER can provide further personalized care to individuals from different cultures and in diverse populations.

References

1. Courtois CA, Ford JD. Treating complex traumatic stress disorders: an evidence-based guide. New York, NY: Guilford Press; 2009. p. 31–58.
2. Arseneault L, Cannon M, Fisher HL, Polanczyk G, Moffitt TE, Caspi A. Childhood trauma and children's emerging psychotic symptoms: a genetically sensitive longitudinal cohort study. Am J Psychiatry. 2011;168(1):65–72.
3. Bendall S, Jackson HJ, Hulbert CA, McGorry PD. Childhood trauma and psychotic disorders: a systematic, critical review of the evidence. Schizophr Bull. 2008;34(3):568–79.
4. Braakman M, Kortmann F, van der Brink W. Validity of post-traumatic stress disorder with secondary features: a review of the evidence. Acta Psychiatr Scand. 2009;119(1):15–24.
5. Croft J, Heron J, Teufel C, et al. Association of trauma type, age of exposure, and frequency in childhood and adolescence with psychotic experiences in early adulthood. JAMA Psychiat. 2018; https://doi.org/10.1001/jamapsychiatry.2018.3155.
6. Scott JG, Cohen D, DiCicco-Bloom B, Miller WL, Stange KC, Crabtree BF. Understanding healing relationships in primary care. Ann Fam Med. 2008;6(4):315–22.
7. Stange KC. The problem of fragmentation and the need for integrative solutions. Ann Fam Med. 2009;7(2):100–3. https://doi.org/10.1370/afm.971.
8. Single Point of Access (SPOA) (n.d.). http://www2.erie.gov/mentalhealth/index.php?q=single-point-access-spoa.
9. Shin LM, Liberzon I. The Neurocircuitry of Fear, Stress and Anxiety Disorders. Neuropsychopharmacology. 2010;35(2010):169–91.
10. Tang YY, Ma YH, Wang J, Fan YX, Feng SG, Lu QL. Short-term meditation training improves attention and self-regulation. Proc Natl Acad Sci U S A. 2007;104:17152–6.

Part III

Training, Policy and Cultural Aspects of TIMBER

6 Cultural Considerations in Applying TIMBER Therapy

6.1 Introduction

Culture can be defined as:

> An integrated pattern of human behavior which includes but is not limited to—thought, communication, languages, beliefs, values, practices, customs, courtesies, rituals, manners of interacting, roles, relationships, and expected behaviors of an ethnic group or social groups whose members are uniquely identifiable by that pattern of human behavior. [1]

Culture influences every aspect of an individual's experience of trauma. This can range from understanding the concept and subjective experience of trauma, its impact, psychological and emotional response, and expression of distress [2]. Culture further influences an individual's resilience in the face of traumatic events, as a strong cultural identity and community supports are determinants in how individuals access help and deal with trauma.

This chapter provides pointers to addressing cultural issues that may arise during the course of therapy, in particular TIMBER therapy. Knowledge of cultural factors help understand an individual's experience of trauma, their resilience, their pathways to care, and their interactions with the mental health system in general and the therapist in particular. It is also important to keep in mind that the philosophy and the framework of TIMBER psychotherapy is in part based on universality of the human experience as enunciated by Gautama Buddha.

Buddha described the *Four Noble Truths* [3, 4] relating to the human experience that transcend differences between human beings such as age, sex, geography, culture, class, and time frame of our existence. These are as below:

1. Suffering is part of human life; it is universal to the "human condition."
2. There is a cause for suffering.
3. Suffering can end.
4. There is a way to end suffering (i.e., the Noble Eightfold Path [4]).

B. Pradhan et al., *TIMBER Psychotherapy*,
https://doi.org/10.1007/978-3-030-20648-2_6

Similarly, Buddha's description of the *five-factor model of the mind* ([5, 6], Chap. 5) *is a universal theory on the human mind* rather than a religious concept. The *five-factor model of the mind* forms one of the foundational cornerstones for the TIMBER therapy. This *Abhidhammic (Theravada Buddhism)* model of mind informs us that mind consists of a bundle of five core domains: *our thoughts, feelings, perceptions, memory, and will.* Otherwise called as the five aggregates (Pali, khandas; Sanskrit, skandhas), these five things are the five contents of the mind. Through these five contents, the mind creates a complete awareness of the objects in our experience. In the process of meditation, by using the mindful detachment and mindful awareness, the role of the meditator is to observe in detached manner the following: how these five aggregates of experience arise or originate in the field of awareness, how they co-create the experience in our awareness by their interdependent actions, and how these experiences change constantly, in an ongoing manner to the point of their eventual dissipation in our field of awareness. The deep philosophies of the mindfulness traditions make us realize that each of these aggregates that constitute the experience is in a state of flux or constant change with respect to itself as well in relation to the other aggregates, i.e., these are impermanent or prone to change constantly, and hence, there is no reason to cling to them or to identify with them. The goal of the meditative praxes described by the early champions like the Buddha and Patanjali was to obtain a better idea (i.e., insight; Pali. *vipassana*) about how these five aggregates function in sequence and in relation to each other to co-create the human experience [7].

Translating these into our current terminology and understanding, TIMBER psychotherapy is about human experience in the context of trauma. Human experience including the trauma experience is a co-creation of the five factors mentioned above that work together: *thoughts, feelings, perceptions, memories and will.* Every individual constantly creates experiences and categorizes them as positive (pleasant/good) or negative (distressing/bad). We all are driven to seek pleasant experiences and avoid unpleasant ones at all costs. Sometimes the choices that we make in life based on this drive to have uninterrupted positive experiences can be the root cause of distress, and this is universal across all cultures. The way to end human distress or suffering is to understand the cause of suffering. We have a skewed understanding of human suffering, and we attribute it to either people or "things" in the environment. However, this does not take into account the role the mind plays in co-creating the experience. Also, what we tend to forget is the transient nature of all human experience. By becoming aware of the role of the mind in co-creating our experience and acknowledging that all experiences that we seek or avoid are temporary and have a short shelf life changes our approach to experiences and moves us on the path of moderation (*The Middle Way of Life*, Dalai Lama [8]), eventually taking us beyond the dualities of positive and negative experiences. The therapist helps the client to come to this understanding and then work on techniques that they can practice at home.

The therapist, by using this approach, puts the therapeutic relationship on a level playing field and thereby reduces the likelihood of various cultural beliefs interfering with engagement and the therapeutic outcome. One essential element of this therapy is that the client actually learns to look at their psychological distress as data or information that they alone have access to. Therefore, they would use the techniques learned to work with this data at a pace they are comfortable with and make a choice to share this data with the therapist as they see fit. This puts every individual, irrespective of their own cultural background or previous experiences in the driver's seat, controlling the gateway to their mind.

6.2 Cultural Diversity Is the Norm

The authors begin with the understanding that every individual has a culture that is unique to them. This may be largely defined by the family, wider community, and societal culture but also influenced by personal experiences. Globalization is broadening multiculturalism and movement of people within and outside their native countries and cultures. This means that individuals who migrate undergo a process of adaptation, or merging of the cultural values and attitudes during the period of prolonged contact with the host culture after immigration, a process called acculturation. As a result of this interaction, there is an inevitable modification of the individuals' attitudes and behaviors. This culture-shifting process is not an abrupt event, and the time period is variable for each individual. The way an individual integrates into a culture is highly individualistic. At one end there are individuals who hold rigidly to their cultural beliefs and values and are cocooned from the rest of the society so that there is no integration. On the other hand most individuals tend to gradually take up values of other culture, a process as described above as acculturation. There tends to be a gradual blending of the two cultures [9], i.e., the culture of the host country and that of their original native country, and sometimes this continues over several generations. It is important for the therapist to be aware of the degree of acculturation as this helps them in making adaptations to enhance engagement. As acculturation is an ongoing process, it is important to understand that an individual's culture is a dynamic concept, and the therapist should be open to updating their understanding of the client in front of them.

Immigration and acculturation are not the only factors that define the dynamism of culture at societal and individual level. Social influence, societal changes, natural disasters, war, national and international policies, and above all an individual's cognitive, emotional, and behavioral responses to these wider changes can be unique, leading to a gradual shift in their personal culture. As an example, while the world has witnessed more diversity due to immigration and free flow of information due to social media, there has also been a recent surge in protectionism and nationalistic tendencies. There is a conflict between integration and territorialism, and this gets amplified during times of economic or political crises, whereby minority cultures can be scapegoated. All the wider societal tensions are played out in an individual's community and their interpretation of life events like grief and trauma. Therefore, cultural diversity is the norm, and understanding this is important for clinicians when practicing with patients.

6.3 Culture and Trauma

Hinton and Lewis-Fernández [10] argue that the cross-cultural validity of any of the definitions of trauma that had been in use since 1980 or, in fact, even their relevance in other cultures is elusive. Most cross-cultural studies have not investigated whether the actual concept of trauma is inherent or innate to cultures other than the Western culture [11]. On the other hand, we know that some cultural groups report higher levels of trauma. We also know that social and ethnocultural responses to traumatic or stressful life events are diverse. Marshall and colleagues [12] used a sample of Hispanic, non-Hispanic Caucasian, and African American survivors of sudden physical injury. They found that the Hispanic group reported higher levels of overall post-traumatic distress and also different patterns of symptoms. A study on victims of the Asian Tsunami from India highlighted that the community collectivized personal trauma, constructed meaning following the disaster using a fatalistic perspective, displayed mourning openly, and employed spiritual beliefs as coping mechanisms [13]. Charak and colleagues [14] studied PTSD (post-traumatic stress disorder) in India and found that the presentation was generally in line with what was described in the West with females showing higher degree of symptoms compared to males. A bibliographic analysis of research in traumatic stress found that 88% of research was in HIC (high-income countries) [15]. When research was published about LMIC (low- and middle-income countries), in 45% of cases no researchers from those countries were co-authors. The authors point out to opportunities for more trauma research in LMIC and equally important is for researchers from those areas to be driving the process.

A biological etiology of the symptoms of post-traumatic stress disorder (PTSD) has been accepted, and therefore it would be fair to assume that the key symptomatology of PTSD would be universal. However, the cultural contexts in which traumatic experiences occur contribute to interpretations of their meaning and responses. As a result, differences have been reported in the symptomatology of PTSD in different cultures. Symptoms like flashbacks vary in their expression across cultural groups, and prevalence rates of distressing dreams are higher in certain cultural groups (reviewed in [16]). Dissociation is an important albeit a less familiar and less studied post-traumatic symptom than flashbacks or depression. It has been defined as the lack of integration of thoughts, feelings, and experiences into the stream of consciousness [17]. Severe dissociation as a component of PTSD could be conceptualized as cognitive avoidance. The use of avoidance is variable in different cultures. In traditional, collectivist cultures, where communities and family's honor is important, avoidance may be an adaptive process following exposure to trauma [18]. In many cultures, somatization of distress is a common manifestation following traumatic experiences [19]. Expression of distress in this way can feel less stigmatizing and possibly more validating.

There is now recognition of the concept of "traumatic psychoses." These are psychotic reactions associated with traumatic experiences (e.g., hallucinations based on the abuser's reappearance) and can occur in people with or without serious mental illnesses [20, 21]. It has been proposed that dissociative experiences, which are relatively common cognitive-emotional reactions in humans [22], are the reason for these experiences. Culture provides the belief system and explanatory model that interprets human emotional and behavioral experiences, including psychotic experiences, both for the sufferer and for the family and community they live within [22, 23].

The context of the trauma and its reporting is often guided by culture. As an example, we know that maltreatment and abuse in children leading to trauma have cross-cultural implications. Immigrant families bring parenting practices and belief systems, sometimes surrounding the use of discipline like corporal punishment. Similarly, cultural norms affect disclosure and reporting of childhood sexual abuse and are variously influenced by religion and global cultural trends [24]. Reporting practices of abuse are noted to be influenced largely by sensitivity, fear, taboo, shame, attitude, acceptable practices and prejudice, community passivity, legal system inadequacies and weaknesses, and the general perceptions and attitudes toward sexual offenses against children [25]. In some cultures, there is a strong belief that girls deserve to be abused because of the way they dress [26]. The response to the trauma in these individuals could amount to shame and guilt including self-blame with symptoms of depression.

Shame and stigma are important cultural considerations following trauma. Fontes [27] has described a number of cultural variables, including responsibility for the abuse, failure to protect, "fate," damaged goods, loss of virginity, predictions of a shameful future, revictimization, and layers of shame that influence this emotion after trauma. In collectivistic cultures, the individual considers shame for themselves and also for their family.

Evidence suggests that culture, in its wider definition, is related and may even dictate rates of exposure to trauma [28]. As an example, refugees experience higher rates of trauma exposure than non-refugees, a status which may be further influenced by variables such as ethnicity [29]. Lesbian, gay, bisexual, and transgender (LGBT) persons experience higher rates of trauma exposure than heterosexual individuals [30], in addition to high rates of normative loss (e.g., family and peer rejection) that LGBT populations face [31]. Female genital mutilation (FGM) is now recognized in many countries due to migration and the victims often presenting to mental health facilities [32]. Female genital mutilations is practiced in areas of East and West Africa extending across to the sub-Saharan region, from Sudan to Senegal along the Nile valley from Egypt down to East Africa, as well as Malaysia, Yemen, India, and Indonesia. Often the reasons given for the continuation of this practice includes religious rites, initiation rite to safeguard virginity, to attenuate sexual desire, aesthetic reasons, and for cure of some ailments [33].

Immigration adds another layer of complexity in understanding the cultural impact of trauma. Migrant families can experience additional trauma through their experiences of racism and discrimination, fear of deportation, socioeconomic status, isolation, loss of family, and community structures. The dynamics between the cultures can vary from peaceful coexistence to outright hostility and overt conflict, leading to variations in traumatic experiences of individuals.

Acculturation trauma or stress can be one of the major stressors precipitating psychosis, particularly when the stress of encountering a different culture and language is sudden or acute (also known as "culture shock"). Other complicating traumatic factors associated with immigration include pre-migratory experiences that led to the emigration (war, natural disaster, terrorism), treacherous emigration journeys (dangerous travel, abuse and victimization, losses of loved ones), and traumatic stressors involved in resettlement (uncertain and insecure residence, loss of contract with family and social supports) [34, 35]. Many studies have pointed to a higher rate of psychotic symptoms and illness among first-generation immigrants.

6.4 Culture and Health Services

Any diagnostic, medical, psychological, or behavioral health intervention should demonstrate effectiveness across different cultures and needs adaptation to make it effective. This implies that services and clinicians need to understand how culture has an impact on the way that interventions are perceived and used. Cultural competence allows clinicians to use precision and specificity in order to be clear when discussing culture and its relevance for therapy. Clinicians should be aware that often the dynamics in wider community plays out in therapeutic settings. To widen the perspective of cultural differences, an understanding of nonethnic-based cultures, such as the gay culture, deaf culture, youth culture, and disability culture, among others, can help a clinician gain appreciation into the presenting issues as well as facilitating the development of therapeutic rapport.

The Diagnostic and Statistical Manual (DSM) V recognizes the importance of cultural factors in psychiatric diagnostic interview and management. The DSM-5 Cultural Formulation Interview (CFI) has been introduced to conduct a culturally competent psychiatric interview. The CFI is a standardized 16-item questionnaire that operationalizes the Outline for Cultural Formulation (OCF), which first appeared in DSM-IV/DSM-IV-TR (American Psychiatric Association 1994, 2000) and was updated in DSM-5. The CFI is intended for use at the initial assessment and provides a useful framework for culturally competent assessment that is both sensitive and responsive to the person's cultural background. The main goal of the OCF is to help clinicians identify cultural contextual factors affecting the patient that are relevant to diagnosis and treatment [36].

Another aspect of ensuring personalized care is recognizing the impact of culture and providing culturally adapted interventions. Evidence suggests that culturally adapted interventions improve outcomes [37]. Our group has developed an evidence-based adaptation framework that has been successfully applied to interventions for different cultural groups [38, 39].

Adaptation in our work has focused on three fundamental areas of delivery, which we refer to as the "Triple-A" principle [38]:

1. Awareness of relevant cultural issues and preparation for therapy: this can be further subdivided into (a) culture and culture-related issues including religion and spirituality, family and community, and language and communication; (b) system and environmental aspects including individual capacity and circumstances, systems of support, services, and help-seeking pathways into care; and (c) cognitive biases and unhelpful beliefs which are directly related to problem and its treatment.
2. Assessment and engagement.
3. Adjustments in therapy.

These areas and subareas are further discussed below in the framework of adaptation. The process of adaptation starts with preparation for the therapy, i.e., preengagement phase as access to therapy and its delivery, and most importantly availability for a given culture is as important as the actual modification of the intervention. The adaptation framework then progresses to engagement and assessment, followed by the adaptation of therapy using relevant cultural aspects.

The authors have developed this adaptation model based on their work, using descriptions initially described by Tseng and colleagues [40] and modifying them. The key principle is that every individual has a unique culture that is influenced by their wider culture and subculture and further developed through unique life experiences. There must be flexibility in applying the culturally adapted therapy, and clinicians should be aware of their own biases, propensity to stereotype when working with people from minority groups. The adaptation framework focuses on the following [41]:

1. Philosophical orientation
2. Practical considerations of societal and health system-related factors
3. Technical adjustments of methods and skills
4. Theoretical adaptations of concepts

Below we briefly describe the framework and how it can be applied by clinicians to TIMBER [41] (Table 6.1).

Table 6.1 Adaptation framework for TIMBER

Framework levels	Areas of adaptation	Subareas of adaptation	Focus of adaptation	Application to TIMBER
Philosophical orientation	Awareness and preparation	Cognitions and beliefs	Beliefs and attributions about illness, health, and health providers (knowledge, beliefs, and expectations about healing and the healers, common presenting complaints, beliefs about illness and its causes, its treatment, treatment providers, therapy, involvement of nonmedical healers) Help-seeking behaviors and pathways into care	Philosophy regarding stress and universality of human experience. This reduces the cultural barriers. In session, focus is on current distressing experiences and cultural understanding for the individual. As a result, prior beliefs and attributions about illness and health are understood
	Levels of acculturation	Migration stress	Oscillation between host culture, culture of origin, and societal culture Intergenerational conflict Cultural identity	Stressors and trauma related to migration. Adaptations are addressed using the five-factor model
	Awareness and preparation/ assessment and engagement	Culture and related factors	Subgroups within areas, e.g., different communities Culture and spirituality Understanding spiritual beliefs of individuals and their families/culture Understanding help-seeking behavior (e.g., spiritual healers, meditating, etc.) **Culture and religion**: There are many subgroups within a religion People who identify with the same religion may have differing views on their faith **Culture sexuality:** Different subcultures within LGBT, e.g., transsexual, bisexual, pansexual LGBT have other issues, e.g., discrimination, anxiety coming out, nonacceptance from family that can add to their mental health	Assessment in TIMBER focuses on the distress client currently experiences and less on the historical aspects. This facilitates engagement as clients find therapy focus as meaningful and relevant Some cultures may need more support and encouragement to practice at home if the belief system is that therapist plays the active role and client's role is more passive
		Language Use of an Interpreter	consider bi-multilingual factor, idioms of distress, images, stories, or metaphors (dependant on upbringing)	

Practical considerations of societal factors	Assessment and engagement	Capacity and circumstances	Societal factors (gender, education, socioeconomic status, reading and writing skills) Immigration factors/policies; health system, local provider reputation, patient experience and satisfaction, levels of **stigma** of mental illness and inequalities, e.g., racism; funding arrangements	
		Stigma and Discrimination		Therapist practice of technique in session with client is powerful antidote for stigma. The cultural implications need to be understood
		Family and friends	Family conflict can affect involvement with services, e.g., lack of understanding or different views regarding mental illness and treatment Family communication—difficult to talk about mental health issues or do not speak about it at all, e.g., feeling family are going to judge Support from family and friends Stigma and family reputation Family relationships are different for each person	TIMBER has wellness component that any family member of client can learn in session. This gives both the client and the family member a common helpful activity to engage in. It also helps to understand the family's cultural perspective, reason for conflict (if any), and support available
	Access and delivery	Capacity and circumstances	System-related issues, e.g.: Not enough support from the government Finding the right help through the mental health system is not easy and can be a long process There is a limit to how much a service can be involved	TIMBER sessions are shorter and fewer and thus suitable in an environment with resource crunch Practice is established in three half hour sessions

(continued)

Table 6.1 (continued)

Framework levels	Areas of adaptation	Subareas of adaptation	Focus of adaptation	Application to TIMBER
Technical adjustments of methods and skills	Assessment and engagement/ adjustment in therapy	Therapeutic alliance	Patient-practitioner relationship: Therapeutic self-disclosure Trust Collaborative empiricism versus Paternalism **Trust:** trust is regarded most important for engagement, especially the ability to disclose. Previous experience with services also affects levels of trust Local idioms of distress, metaphors/stories, etc.	Therapist describes the five-factor model of mind as common to therapist as well as client thereby making the relationship even Therapist own experience with wellness model, and self-disclosure about it helps client engagement Therapist practices with client in session thereby reducing stigma and modeling right practice Model is made to fit the individuals experience and not the other way round in a collaborative empirical manner
	Helping make sense	Cultural formulation	Other events that came before symptoms—experiences, e.g., trauma	Understanding the context and interpretation of trauma including attributions and supports
Theoretical modifications of concepts	Western vs. eastern traditional views Family structure and goals Role of religion and spirituality and sexuality		Prayer can be helpful to some Understanding individual's personal and cultural values and incorporating these in their support	
	Relapse prevention/ endings			
	Individualist/ collectivist concepts Personality development Therapeutic stance	Individual goals Authoritative (prescriptive) vs. collaborative	Understanding patient's perspective and world view People have different opinions, personalities, and experiences Needs are constantly changing, depending on the stage an individual is at	Therapy allows the client to understand their distress, cause of suffering and how this is influenced by culture

6.5 Conclusions

Culture plays a significant role in how trauma is perceived and dealt with by the individual, the family, and the wider community. Therapists should be aware of the role of cultural factors in their client's presentation. The five-factor model of the mind provides a common framework to deal with any type of human experience as it recognizes that universality of human experience. The TIMBER technique is designed to break the usual cultural barriers, and the therapy places the client and therapist on the same footing. The therapist's own practice and ability to access the meditative state of their mind facilitates the client to get to the same meditative state while in session. This synchrony of mental states is the best way to overcome the existing cultural barriers.

References

1. National Center for Cultural Competence (2004). Georgetown University Center for Child and Human Development. http://gucchd.georgetown.edu/nccc.
2. Kirmayer LJ, Sartorius N. Cultural models and somatic syndromes. Psychosom Med. 2007;69:832–40.
3. Analayo B. Satipatthana: the direct path to realization. Birmingham: Windhorse Publications; 2003.
4. Nyanamoli B. The path of purification (*Visuddhimagga*). Kandy: Buddhist Publication Society; 1975.
5. Pradhan BK. Yoga and mindfulness based cognitive therapy: a clinical guide. Berlin: Springer; 2014.
6. Pradhan BK, Pinninti NR, Rathod S. Brief interventions for psychosis: a clinical compendium. Switzerland: Springer Publishers; 2016.
7. Pradhan BK, Gogineni RR, Sharma S. Mind, Mindfulness, and the Social Brain: Psychobiological Understandings and Implications. Ind J Soc Psychiatr. 2018;34(4):313–22.
8. Lama D. The middle way: faith grounded in reason (trans: Jinpa T). Boston: Wisdom Publications; 2009.
9. Garcia G, Zea C, (1997). Psychological interventions and research with Latino populations. Allyn & Bacon Boston.
10. Hinton DE, Lewis-Fernández R. The cross-cultural validity of post-traumatic stress disorder: implications for DSM-5. Depress Anxiety. 2011;28:1–19. https://doi.org/10.1002/da.20753.
11. Caspi, Y., Ghafoori, B., Smith, S., and Contractor, A., on behalf of the Diversity and Cultural Competency SIG. (2013). On the Importance of Considering Culture When Defining Trauma. Stresspoints.
12. Marshall GN, Schell TL, Miles JN. Ethnic differences in post traumatic distress: Hispanics' symptoms differ in kind and degree. J Consult Clin Psychol. 2009;77(6):1169–78.
13. Rajkumar AP, Premkumar TS, Tharyan P. Coping with the Asian tsunami: Perspectives from Tamil Nadu, India on the determinants of resilience in the face of adversity. Soc Sci Med. 2008;67:844–53.
14. Charak R, Armour C, Elklit A, Angmo D, Elhai JD, Koot HM. Factor structure of PTSD, and relation with gender in trauma survivors from India. Eur J Psychotraumatol. 2014;5(1).
15. Fodor KE, Unterhitzenberger J, Chou C, Kartal D, Leister S, Milosavljevic M, et al. Is traumatic stress research global? A bibliometric analysis. Eur J Psychotraumatol. 2014;5:23269. https://doi.org/10.3402/ejpt.v5.23269.
16. Hinton DE, Lewis-Fernández R. The cross-cultural validity of posttraumatic stress disorder: Implications for DSM-V. Depress Anxiety. 2010;0:1–19. https://doi.org/10.1002/da.20753.
17. Bernstein EM, Putnam FW. Development, reliability, and validity of a dissociation scale. J Nerv Ment Dis. 1986;174:727–35.

18. Elsass P. Individual and collective traumatic memories: A qualitative study of post-traumatic stress disorder symptoms in two Latin American localities. Transcult Psychiatry. 2001;38(3):306–16. https://doi.org/10.1177/136346150103800302.
19. Kleinman A. Depression, somatization and the new cross-cultural psychiatry. Soc Sci Med. 1977;11(1):3–10.
20. Kingdon DG, Turkington D. Cognitive-behavioral therapy of schizophrenia: Guilford Publications; 2005. p. 40–41 and 52-53.
21. Rathod S, Irfan M, Bhargava R, et al. Multinational comparative cross-sectional survey of views of medical students about acceptable terminology and subgroups in schizophrenia. BMJ Open. 2018;8:e021461. https://doi.org/10.1136/bmjopen-2017-021461.
22. Castillo RJ. Trance, functional psychosis, and culture. Psychiatry. 2003;66:9–21.
23. Spiegel J. Transactions: the interplay between individual, family, and society. New York: Science House; 1971.
24. Shafe S, Hutchinson G. Child sexual abuse and continuous influence of cultural practices: a review. West Indian Med J. 2014;63(6):634–7.
25. Kisanga F, Nystrom L, Hogam N, Emmelin M. Child sexual abuse: common concern in urban Tanzania. J Child Sex Abuse. 2011;20:196–217.
26. Lalor K. Child sexual abuse in Tanzania and Kenya. Child Abuse Negl. 2004;28(8):833–44.
27. Fontes LA. Child abuse and culture: working with diverse families. New York: Guildford; 2005.
28. Roberts AL, Gilman SE, Breslau J, Breslau N, Koenen KC. Race/ethnic differences in exposure to traumatic events, development of post-traumatic stress disorder, and treatment-seeking for post-traumatic stress disorder in the United States. Psychol Med. 2011;41:71–83. https://doi.org/10.1017/S0033291710000401.
29. Keller A, Lhewa D, Rosenfeld B, Sachs E, Aladjem A, Cohen I, Smith H, Porterfield K. Traumatic experiences and psychological distress in an urban refugee population seeking treatment services. J Nerv Ment Dis. 2006;194:188–94.
30. Brown LS, Pantalone D. Lesbian, gay, bisexual and transgender issues in trauma psychology: a topic comes out of the closet. Traumatology. 2011;17:1–3.
31. Brown LS. Sexuality, lies, and loss: lesbian, gay, and bisexual perspectives on trauma. J Trauma Prac. 2003;2:55–68.
32. McClellan J, Adams J, Douglas D, McCurry C, Storck M. Clinical characteristics related to severity of sexual abuse: a study of seriously mentally ill youth. Child Abuse Negl. 1995;19(10):1245–54.
33. Karim M, Ammar R. Female circumcision and sexual desire. Cairo: Ain Shams University Press; 1985.
34. Bhugra D. Migration and mental health. Acta Psychiat Scand. 2004;109(4):243–58.
35. Rothe E, Tzuang D, Pumariega AJ. Acculturation, development, and adaptation. Child Adolesc Psychiatr Clin N Am. 2010;19(4):681–96.
36. Mezzich JE, Carraci G, Fabrega H, Kir-mayer LJ. Cultural formulation guidelines. Transcult Psychiatry. 2009;46:383–405.
37. Rathod S, Giga L, Degnan A, et al. The current status of culturally adapted mental health interventions: a practice-focused review of meta=analysis. Neuropsychiatr Dis Treat. 2017;13: 1–14.
38. Naeem F, Phiri P, Nasar A, Gerada A, Munshi T, Ayub M, Rathod S. An evidence-based framework for cultural adaptation of Cognitive Behaviour Therapy: Process, methodology and foci of adaptation. World Cult Psych Res Review. 2016;11(1/2):61–70.
39. Rathod S, Phiri P, Harris S, Underwood C, Thagadur M, Padmanabi U, Kingdon D. Cognitive behaviour therapy for psychosis can be adapted for minority ethnic groups: a randomised controlled trial. Schizophr Res. 2013;143(2–3):319–26.
40. Tseng WS, Chang SC, Nishizono M, editors. Asian culture and psychotherapy: implications for east and west. Honolulu: University of Hawaii Press; 2005.
41. Rathod, et al. Cultural Adaptation of CBT for Serious Mental illness: a guide for training and practice. Hoboken: Wiley – Blackwell; 2015.

7 Therapist Training on TIMBER and Policy Implications

7.1 Current Healthcare System Globally

Healthcare systems are dynamic and have to constantly change and evolve based on the prevailing forces impacting upon the country or community where care is delivered. The forces that broadly impact healthcare systems are the economic platforms, health needs of populations, epidemics, advancements in the diagnostics and therapeutics, and the changing attitudes and expectations of the consumers of healthcare. In addition, the global world we are in these days makes it quite easy for the flow of healthcare advancements globally that in turn influences the attitudes and expectations of the populations around the world. Let us take a bird's eye view of the current environment in the world to look at some macro forces that are universal to all countries and then some specific circumstances relevant for individual countries.

With respect to healthcare, some of the universal macro forces are as below:

(a) Health of individuals is a universal human right as espoused by UN charter of human rights [1]. All sovereign nations espouse the importance of the health of their population though the resources available for each of the countries to spend on health vary widely. The OECD (Organization for Economic Co-operation and Development) is a group of 30 industrialized countries that spend 7% of their GDP on health in 2013, while at the top end, United States spends 17% of GDP on health [2, 3].
(b) The expectations of people for better health will continue to rise as a result of the free flow of information through social media and better informed public. Now it is very easy for anyone with access to the Internet to compare the health status of different nations of the world with a few clicks.
(c) Healthcare costs will continue to rise as a result of new medications, technologies, and treatments as well as increase in life span of individuals. However, the healthcare budget in any country is finite, and it will be increasingly difficult to absorb the cost of new treatments.

B. Pradhan et al., *TIMBER Psychotherapy*,
https://doi.org/10.1007/978-3-030-20648-2_7

(d) The allocation of resources to healthcare is significantly affected by other priorities of the country such as defense. In conflict-torn regions, security and defense budget trumps healthcare needs, and population health suffers when there is a conflict.

These macro forces trigger every country to come up with its own unique system to balance the *three pillars of healthcare delivery system*: *access, quality, and cost.* As a general rule it is easier to improve one of the three pillars such as quality or access at one time and is not possible to improve all three. So, when quality services are provided and access to these services is improved, then it is not always possible to keep the costs lower in the short term. In order to reduce the cost while improving the quality of services and access, these systems need a paradigm shift in how we as individuals and nations approach health and illnesses.

Currently healthcare is based on a curative model with individuals having access to healthcare system when they are ill, while the preventive care is at best patchy: thus, making the health promotion-related activities quite meager. The individuals are primarily responsible for their own health, and when there is a problem, they access the healthcare system. The focus of healthcare systems is diagnosis and treatment of the medical conditions, while limited attention is paid to the broad social context of the individual within which these health problems arise. The health conditions are treated through various interventions, while health promotion, prevention, and self-management are areas that are neglected as effective strategies in health [4].

A paradigm shift that we need is to make healthcare systems responsible for wellness and health maintenance as well rather than just focusing on diagnosis and treatment of specific medical conditions for these individuals. The WHO encouraged countries to see primary health as a means to care for the entire person and all their healthcare needs through the lifetime including wellness promotion, prevention, management of chronic conditions, and palliative care [5]. However, the health of a defined population is significantly impacted by social determinants, and hence healthcare needs have to be addressed in conjunction with social needs. When healthcare needs are addressed by integrating them with social needs such as housing, income support, nutrition support, care coordination, and community outreach, there are better healthcare outcomes as well as reduction in healthcare spending [6].

Treatment for some severely mentally ill can last for a lifetime, heightening concerns about long-term costs [7]. Self-management refers to "the ability of the individual, in conjunction with family, community, and healthcare professionals, to manage symptoms, treatments, lifestyle changes, and psychosocial, cultural, and spiritual consequences of health conditions" ([8], p. 261). Shifting responsibility of some aspects of health management to patients requires a change in societal, political, and system cultures. Evidence suggests that healthcare practitioners are still not necessarily well equipped to promote self-management given a relative lack of training in self-management approaches [9]. MD-Value in Prevention (MDVIP) is a network of affiliated primary care physicians in the United States who utilize a model of healthcare delivery based on an augmented physician-patient relationship and focused on personalized preventive healthcare. MDVIP members experienced reduced utilization of emergency room and urgent care services, and there was overall reduction in cost of providing service [10]. This study showed that the additional cost in physician time in building and maintaining relationship with patients is more than paid for in improved quality while lowering the overall costs to the system.

7.2 High- and Middle-Income Countries (HMIC)

Across the HMIC, there is a drive to move the mental healthcare from the state institutions and asylums to community settings through the establishment of community mental health centers (CMHCs) and teams (CMHTs). Despite this and the evidence of efficacy, psychosocial interventions are shown to be highly underutilized in the treatment of illnesses such as schizophrenia [11].

The public as well as personal healthcare costs in the United States have been progressively rising well above the rate of inflation and currently stand at 17% of the gross domestic product (GDP) [12]. All HMIC have been combating escalating healthcare costs through a variety of cost containing mechanisms [13]. In the United States while the costs were high, there were significant problems in healthcare delivery, and outcomes with 16% of population had no health insurance, and healthcare in the United States was poorer than most countries in Organization of Economic Development (OECD). Among 34 OECD countries between 1990 and 2010, the United States rank for the age-standardized death rate went down from 18th to 27th, for life expectancy at birth from 20th to 27th, and for health-adjusted life expectancy (HALE) from 14th to 26th [14]. In the United States, the affordable care act addressed some of the long-standing issues in US healthcare by reducing uninsured from 16 to 9.1%, improving access to care, and changing part of payment system to one based on quality of care and outcomes [15]. Despite these improvements, the challenges facing US healthcare remain. One of the challenges is significant opposition to affordable care health and ongoing political efforts to repeal affordable care and turn back the clock. The opioid epidemic is the single more important healthcare crisis in the United States taking the lives of 174 every day in the United States, and this death toll comprises of mostly young people. Even though the focus is on opiates, deaths are from various drugs, and drug overdose deaths have been increasing exponentially for the past 38 years in epidemic proportions [16].

In the United Kingdom, new models of care are being developed based on population health and illness as it is widely acknowledged that the current system of care provided by the National Health Service (NHS) will not be able to meet the needs of an aging population and rising long-term conditions. For example, in 2016 the United Kingdom launched the National Access and Waiting Time Standard (AWTS) program that aims to reduce the duration of untreated psychosis by early detection and appropriate and timely treatment. In the United Kingdom, the National Institute for Health and Care Excellence (NICE) provides the evidence-based quality standards and has initiated the development and implementation of the integrated care pathways (ICPs) with a view to providing early access, holistic physical and mental healthcare, and improved outcomes. ICPs are important because they improve the quality of care and serve to reduce unnecessary variations in patient care and outcomes. The ICPs can also be used as a tool to implement and incorporate local and national guidelines into everyday practice, manage clinical risk, and meet the requirements of clinical governance. These new models of care aim to improve coordination of services, provide more proactive support for the health needs of populations and individuals, and move care out of hospital where appropriate. There is national support (such as King's Fund) to achieve this ambition.

The European healthcare system is complex and changing in response to austerity. Stuckler et al. [17] discuss the "social risk effect" through increasing poverty, homelessness, and unemployment and the "healthcare effect" through reductions in services. Austerity has a significant impact on a population's mental health [17]. A multicountry study using longitudinal data from health and retirement surveys in the United States and 13 EU countries found that job loss among 50–64-year-olds, particularly when due to firm closure, was associated with a 28% increase in depressive symptoms in the United States and of 8% in Europe [18]. Evidence from many countries like Australia, Spain, and Ireland confirms the impact of austerity on depression [19].

7.3 Low- and Middle-Income Countries (LMIC)

Over 80% of people suffering from mental disorders are residing in LMICs, with mental illness and substance abuse disorders presenting as an important cause of disease burden, accounting for 8.8% and 16.6% of the total burden of disease in low-income and lower middle-income countries, respectively [5]. Singla et al. [20] did a systematic review of psychological treatments delivered by non-specific providers in LMIC. They found that treatments were commonly delivered by community health workers or peers in primary care or community settings; they usually were delivered with fewer than ten sessions over 2–3 months in an individual, face-to-face format. Treatments included common elements, such as non-specific engagement and specific domains of behavioral, interpersonal, emotional, and cognitive elements. The pooled effect size was 0.49 (95% confidence interval = 0.36-0.62), favoring intervention conditions. They concluded that psychological treatments—comprising a parsimonious set of common elements and delivered by a low-cost, widely available human resource—have moderate to strong effects in reducing the burden of common mental disorders [20]. Rathod et al. [21] have discussed the key challenges and opportunities in LMICs when delivering mental health services that meet the needs of their populations, further making recommendations on how future development and delivery of mental healthcare in LMICs can be informed and influenced by evidence and successful service models [21].

The challenges of low- and middle-income countries are different and include significant limitation of skilled professionals to treat individuals with mental health conditions and sequelae of trauma. The challenges also offer innovative opportunities. For example, lay public with interest in mental health can be trained to successfully deliver psychological interventions. This approach was used for treating alcoholism and depression in primary care settings in rural India. The outcome was that individuals who received motivational interview and CBT (cognitive behavioral therapy)-based culturally adapted interventions showed significantly better outcomes than the control group [22]. One strength of the LMIC is a stronger social fabric with families and communities having more ties with mentally ill individuals and willing to take many of the tasks that the social workers or therapists do in high-income countries.

7.4 Trauma and Health

The faster mode of transportation and near ubiquitous use of social media has made the world a much smaller place, and individuals are bombarded by traumatic news either from natural disasters or man-made events. We are now in a world where disaster news is delivered to our phones within minutes of something happening in the world. The result is that exposure to vicarious trauma is much higher now and places all individuals at risk for vicarious traumatic stress and other trauma-related disorders. There is growing evidence that adversity and trauma particularly that experienced during childhood are associated with poor physical and psychological health as well as increased morbidity and mortality. Felitti et al. [23] found that people who had experienced four or more categories of childhood adversity and trauma had 4- to 12-fold increased health risks for alcoholism, drug abuse, depression, and suicide attempts compared to those who had none. The mediators of adverse effects are high-risk health-related behaviors such as smoking, physical inactivity, and having 50 or more sexual partners [23]. There is a relationship between number of categories of adverse childhood exposures and a variety of diseases in adult population including ischemic heart disease, cancer, chronic lung disease, skeletal fractures, and liver disease. In addition to this, immigration is associated with significant trauma particularly when it is involuntary and people have to immigrate due to persecution and/or threats to their life. Recently there has been an increase in nationalistic sentiment in many parts of the world, and there is a backlash against immigrants leading to more barriers for immigration and a risk of being traumatized in the new country. Despite the increased exposure to trauma in many individuals and communities and the adverse impact of trauma, there is not adequate attention paid in addressing trauma in a comprehensive manner. However, some forward-looking organizations are taking the initiative to incorporate trauma awareness and training and thereby trying to become trauma-informed organizations.

A trauma-informed organization (TIO) trains its workforce to understand the critical role the trauma plays in the following aspects:

(a) Delaying or distorting normal psychological development of children
(b) Causing psychological distress and various psychiatric illnesses
(c) Barriers that prior trauma places in effective engagement of clients

It is also recognized that staff may come with history of trauma or experience vicarious trauma through their work. Staff trauma is normalized, and systems are in place to support staff in dealing with trauma and its health impacts. TIO places clients and their healthcare experience front and center in both clinical and administrative decisions, and the services are adapted based on ongoing direct data of clients experience and outcome. The organization that the second author works for (Oaks Integrated Care in New Jersey, USA) is a trauma-informed organization that has a standardized trauma training program for all its staff including those with administrative and support role functions. This training is highly valued by staff, and ongoing efforts are to view care through the lenses of trauma.

7.5 Importance of Early Intervention

As discussed earlier, the current healthcare model focusses on illness rather than prevention and early detection. We will demonstrate the need for early intervention in trauma using the example of psychosis. The outlook for psychosis is worse when there is a lag between onset of psychotic symptoms and obtaining help, termed as duration of untreated psychosis (DUP). DUP is considered to be the strongest predictor of symptom severity and prognosis [24, 25]. Longer durations of untreated psychosis can occur due to client-related or service-related factors or both. Client-related factors could be attributable to an inability to recognize early symptoms or due to the illness itself such as poor insight, due to social and emotional withdrawal [26], or due to cultural values systems like attributions to illness and help-seeking pathways into care [27, 28]. The UK government strategy "No health without mental health" acknowledged that more must be done to address the disparity in care for people experiencing psychosis. It highlighted the importance of prevention, early detection, and support for evidence-based models such as early intervention in psychosis (EIP) services. As mentioned before, the National Access and Waiting Time (AWTS) standard for psychosis was announced in the United Kingdom which set the standard requirement from 1 April 2016; more than 50% of people experiencing first episode psychosis should commence a NICE-recommended package of care within 2 weeks of referral. These policy initiatives recognize the impact of early intervention [29].

The Dutch Early Detection Intervention Evaluation (EDIE) trial is another important study done in the Netherlands on individuals who are ultrahigh risk for psychosis [30]. In this study, 196 patients at ultrahigh risk (UHR) of psychosis at 6 sites in the Netherlands were randomized to treatment as usual (TAU) or TAU plus cognitive behavior therapy (CBT) of 26 sessions in the first 6 months. UHR is defined as a group of patients with either a family history of psychosis or significant impairments in cognition or social and occupational functioning that has not yet risen to the level of clinical psychosis. The intervention was to prevent conversion to psychosis, and the follow-up was for 4 years. The number of participants converting to psychosis in the CBT plus TAU was 12 at 4-year follow-up, and it was 22 for

TAU group. The researchers noted that this rate of conversion continues to represent a significantly better outcome for the CBT group over 4 years. Moreover, the number of days to transition to psychosis was significantly higher in the CBT group (1322.45 days) compared with the TAU group (1188.91 days). In the best interest of patients, it is important to make early detection/therapeutic intervention a major priority because it is our best opportunity to improve the life course in persons vulnerable to distressing conditions. The current emphasis on first psychotic episode is a good template for other conditions including trauma.

7.6 Bringing the Different Teams Together (Integrated Care)

Individuals with serious mental illnesses have a variety of needs that can be grouped under four headings of (a) behavioral healthcare needs, (b) addiction needs, (c) physical health needs, and (d) social service needs. Usually multiple teams address these various needs in different programs which do not talk to each other and without responsibility of coordinating all the needs being with any one. The result is that client's experience of care is burdensome, fragmented, lacking continuity, and at times outright traumatizing. Mohammed et al. in a systematic review presented ten quality measures that are important from patient perspective, and these are communication, access, shared decision making, provider knowledge and skills, physical environment, patient education, electronic medical record, pain control, discharge process, and preventive services [31]. In order to improve client experience of care, organizations should develop a client-centered philosophy of care that drives the attitudes and decision making process of all staff in the organization. An example of philosophy of care from the second author is in appendix one. In addition, healthcare processes can be complex, opaque, and not easy to navigate particularly for individuals who are distressed. This can be addressed by identifying or designating an individual or a team to help coordinate the different aspects of care and facilitate the individuals' progress through the care system. In addition, there should be a mechanism in place to get ongoing feedback from the clients about their experience of the services and work with them collaboratively to solve any issues.

7.7 Impact of Trauma on Staff

From the staff perspective, behavioral healthcare provision is becoming more stressful with high levels of burnout. This is in part related to the vicarious trauma that individuals experience during the course of their work. In a meta-analysis of 33 studies, O′Connor and colleagues reported that average mental health staff shows high levels of emotional exhaustion and moderate levels of depersonalization but retain reasonable levels of personal accomplishment. Work-related factors such as workload and relationships at work are key determinants for burnout, while role clarity, a sense of professional autonomy, a sense of being fairly treated, and access to regular clinical supervision appear to be protective [32]. Similarly, in a review of literature, Johnson et al. reported that staff in mental healthcare report poorer well-being than staff in other healthcare sectors. Poorer well-being and higher burnout are associated with poorer quality and safety of patient care, higher absenteeism, and higher turnover rates. Interventions targeted to help staff burnout have been shown to be successful. [33]. As described before, TIMBER has a wellness component, the *standardized meditation program* (StaMP), which has been shown to be well received by staff and reported by staff to be effective in reducing their stress levels and increasing a sense of well-being and accomplishment at work [34]. In the second author's organization, the counselors as well as case managers who work in partial hospitalization program and community have been trained in the StaMP model and encouraged to incorporate the practice into their routine. In addition to personal benefits, all members of the mental healthcare team that comes in contact with the client can reinforce the practice of TIMBER and also engage in practice with clients in office-based as well as in community settings.

7.8 Addressing the Fragmented Care

Different approaches and innovations are trying to address the issue of fragmented care. The 5-year forward view in the United Kingdom (NHS England) recommends development of standardized care pathways for every major mental health condition. Evidenced-based integrated pathways provide a standardized framework for good clinical practice, reduce variation in care, and have improved outcomes for patients through providing timely access and intervention. Standardized pathways improve quality by improving multidisciplinary communication with different care agencies using care planning and improve patient satisfaction [35]. Rathod et al. [36] have developed an integrated care pathway TRIumPH (*Treatment and Recovery In PsycHosis*) for psychosis that prescribes time frames around different aspects of care for people experiencing the first episode psychosis. TRIumPH was established to promote early intervention and good clinical practice and reduce variation in care. This allows an integrated approach to care in a timely manner. Evaluation of the TRIumPH has shown positive results (Rathod et al., unpublished data). Availability of therapies like TIMBER in a timely way could improve long-term outcomes.

Another positive change occurring in behavioral health is the incorporation of peers in work force. There are 42 states that have provisions for peer providers for mental illness and 11 states that allow SUD peer providers [37]. Peers are also called as experts by experience, and they bring about a unique perspective and experience that is invaluable for engaging clients, engendering hope, and guiding individuals toward recovery. Clients are far more likely to reach out to peers in the face of impending crisis, thereby allowing the peer and thereby the mental system of care to intervene and prevent a full-blown crisis [38].

7.9 CCBHCs: Future of Integrated System of Care for the United States

CCBHCs were created through Section 223 of the Protecting Access to Medicare Act [39], which established a demonstration program based on the Excellence in Mental Health Act. The Excellence in Mental Health Act demonstration program also known as the Excellence Act or the Section 223 demonstration program is a 2-year, eight-state initiative to expand Americans' access to mental health and addiction care in community-based settings. There was paradigm shift in funding wherein enhanced funding was approved based on anticipated costs. CCBHCs were made responsible for directly providing (or contracting with partner organizations to provide) nine required types of services, with an emphasis on the provision of 24-hour crisis care, utilization of evidence-based practices, care coordination, and integration with physical healthcare. The financial security of cost-based reimbursement meant that the energies of the organizations were entirely devoted to creating system of care that is outcome focused as opposed to spending time trying to survive fiscally. In December 2016 the Substance Abuse and Mental Health Services Administration announced the selection of the eight participating states: Minnesota, Missouri, Nevada, New Jersey, New York, Oklahoma, Oregon, and Pennsylvania [40].

Survey data of CCBHCs: The CCBHCs have improved access by providing services such as ambulatory detoxification and medication-assisted treatment where no services existed, reduced wait times for existing services thereby improving client engagement, and improved integration of behavioral health, addictions, and physical health while meeting the social needs of the individuals. The survey results are robust enough that this could become the template for changing the existing system of providing behavioral healthcare.

CCBHCs give individual organizations the ability to adapt services based on the needs of the community they serve without the concern of financial jeopardy. The current limitations of care provision for individuals with all psychological consequences of trauma are (a) lack of comprehensive evaluation of trauma and its impact on the lives of individuals, (b) services which can be time limited thereby giving limited time to enable individuals to deal trauma, (c) existing payment systems not allowing combination of services such as addiction and trauma services, (d) lack of trained trauma therapists, and (e) limitations of existing therapies. Below we describe the process for training the therapists on TIMBER.

7.10 Module for Training the Professionals on the TIMBER Psychotherapy

TIMBER therapy is administered on an outpatient basis by a trained therapist after the therapist has been sufficiently trained in its methodology and application in five sequential steps as detailed below:

1. Training on the conceptual foundation of TIMBER and its methodology
2. Observation of the standardized meditation training of clients as well as the application of TIMBER interventions in real time in disorder specific and customized ways
3. Establishing in the trainee therapist the personal practice of meditation
4. Trainee therapist to apply TIMBER interventions on 2–3 practice cases in standardized ways and collect the data on 3–4 sessions
5. Trainee therapist to present the collected data (written and/or audiovisual) on these 2–3 cases and get supervisory support from Dr. Pradhan or an expert on TIMBER via in-person session or phone/videoconferencing

The training of the therapists on conceptual foundation of TIMBER and its methodology is usually done over a 3-hour didactic session using oral presentation, audiovisual study materials, and interactive simulations and discussions. The trainee will be provided access to videos on TIMBER done by Drs. Pradhan and Pinninti through a link that is provided as part of training. Trainee therapists are encouraged to observe the standardized meditation training of clients as well as the application of TIMBER interventions in real time in disorder-specific and customized ways in Dr. Pradhan's clinic. The trainee therapist is encouraged to maintain personal practice of meditation (the Wellness version of TIMBER method) for managing personal stress, improving quality of life, and providing experiential and hands-on knowledge to the clients of the meditative practice experience. After establishing the conceptual clarity on TIMBER from the didactics and completing 3–4 weeks of personal practice, usually watching the execution of these interventions over three to four sessions (30 to 45-min each) is enough for the trainee therapist to begin the application on clients.

Once these three steps are completed, the trainee therapist is encouraged to collect data on 2–3 practice cases and present these cases for supervision to Dr. Pradhan. When the trainee therapist has successfully gone through the above five steps ((1) to (5)), he or she can carry out TIMBER interventions independently with use of booster training sessions as needed. As of December 2018, Dr. Pradhan has successfully trained six therapists (four licensed clinical social workers, LCSWs, and two clinical psychologists), five resident physicians (three residents in psychiatry and one resident in pediatrics, all in their third year of training), and one third year medical student in TIMBER therapy. All of them are able to independently apply the TIMBER interventions to clients with chronic PTSD, depression, and traumatic psychosis.

Clinical settings such as the CCBHCs remain an ideal place to incorporate TIMBER psychotherapy to help individuals deal with trauma. As mentioned before, the *standardized meditation program* (StaMP) which is the wellness component of the TIMBER psychotherapy has been shown to be well received by staff and reported by staff to be effective in reducing their stress levels and increasing a sense of well-being and accomplishment at work [34]. In addition to personal benefits, all members of the mental healthcare team that come in contact with the client can reinforce the practice of TIMBER and also engage in practice with clients in office-based as well as in community settings.

The following is a suggested process that can be incorporated in a CCBHC model. All individuals undergo a comprehensive assessment of their experience of trauma throughout their life course. Then individuals are risk stratified based on the degree of trauma and the impact of trauma on the four components that make up their health and quality of life: physical health needs, behavioral health needs, addiction needs, and social needs. Then services are matched to the more prevalent needs of the individual and for high-risk population. High-risk individuals are provided with a navigator or care coordinator who helps them navigate through the various stages of their recovery journey. All staff in the entire CCBHC including administrative staff should be trained on the *standardized meditation program* (StaMP) which is the wellness component of the TIMBER psychotherapy. Such training benefits in several ways. StaMP helps all staff to deal with the stress inherent in their jobs as well and reduce the likelihood of burnout. Personal experience of wellness model helps the staff to discuss this with clients and also to practice with them. Some of the staff see clients in their natural environments, and by helping them and practicing with them in their natural environment, client distress can be reduced and mindfulness-based skills strengthened. Finally the training gives all staff a common vocabulary as well as shared experience that helps in communicating about client recovery in a consistent manner. While all staff are trained in StaMP, therapists get advanced training to be able to teach the clients the illness aspect of TIMBER and would provide therapy as detailed in Chap. 6. For the leadership of the organization, StaMP- and TIMBER-based interventions can be brought into the supervision to help staff perform optimally while maintaining their emotional health.

7.11 Future Directions for Research

There are several areas in which future research can inform the implementation of TIMBER in routine clinical settings. It is important to find the place of TIMBER for pathways of care for individuals with trauma-induced psychiatric conditions. For this randomized controlled trials, comparing TIMBER with other evidence-based interventions is needed. Another area that needs study is the training of adequate number of staff to being able to provide TIMBER to all clients who suffer from trauma-related conditions of PTSD, treatment-resistant depression, and traumatic psychosis. This is particularly important for clients in remote and rural areas without access to trained therapist. Toward this end, the first author has successfully pioneered the provision of TIMBER via videoconferencing for clients located in rural areas [41]. Videoconferencing also needs to be studied to train staff in TIMBER model so that skill building for workforce can be facilitated. Based on clinical experience of the authors and their ongoing studies, TIMBER has the potential to help other condition such as addictive disorders, borderline personality disorder. In conditions such as addictive disorder, borderline personality disorder, and chronic pain, TIMBER needs to be studied more as a stand-alone therapy or in combination with other therapeutic modalities such as ketamine infusion, propranolol, and transcranial magnetic stimulation (TMS) [42]. Another area for further study is other biomarkers in addition to plasma D-serine such as autonomic response biomarkers (EEG, heart rate variability, and breath pattern analysis) [43].

7.12 Conclusion

This book lays out the theoretical frame work, evidence base for new treatment TIMBER for trauma and trauma-related psychiatric conditions of PTSD, treatment-resistant depression, and traumatic psychosis. TIMBER with its wellness component effectively addresses the stress and burnout in staff as well as helps in building therapeutic relationship effectively. The evidence for D-serine as a biomarker for TIMBER is exciting and very promising. By studying the efficacy and effectiveness in further randomized controlled trials, the place of TIMBER in care pathways of individuals due to psychiatric sequelae of trauma can be delineated.

References

1. Castillo CHM, Garrafa V, Cunha T, Hellmann F. Access to health care as a human right in international policy: critical reflections and contemporary challenges. Cien Saude Colet. 2017;22(7):2151–60. https://doi.org/10.1590/1413-81232017227.04472017.
2. de la Maisonneuve C, Oliveira MJ. (2013). A Projection Method for Public Health and Long Term Care Expenditures: OECD Economics Department Working Paper no 1048. https://read.oecd-ilibrary.org/economics/a-projection-method-for-public-health-and-long-term-care-expenditures_5k44v53w5w47-en#page1.
3. Moses H 3rd, Matheson DH, Dorsey ER, George BP, Sadoff D, Yoshimura S. The anatomy of health care in the United States. JAMA. 2013;310(18):1947–63. https://doi.org/10.1001/jama.2013.281425.
4. Madsen W. Early 20th century conceptualization of health promotion. Health Promot Int. 2017;32(6):1041–7. https://doi.org/10.1093/heapro/daw039.
5. WHO. (2008). World Health Organization. The global burden of disease; accessed on 012119. https://www.who.int/primary-health/en/.
6. Taylor LA, Tan AX, Coyle CE, Ndumele C, Rogan E, Canavan M, et al. Leveraging the social determinants of health: what works? PLoS One. 2016;11(8):e0160217. https://doi.org/10.1371/journal.pone.0160217.
7. Clark RE, Samnaliev M. Psychosocial treatment in the 21st century. Int J Law Psychiatry. 2005;28(5):532–44.
8. Richard AA, Shea K. Delineation of self-care and associated concepts. J Nurs Scholarsh. 2011;43(3):255–64. https://doi.org/10.1111/j.1547-5069.2011.01404.x.
9. Lake AJ, Staiger PK. Seeking the views of health professionals on translating chronic disease self-management models into practice. Patient Educ Couns. 2010;79(1):62–8.
10. Musich S, Wang S, Hawkins K, Klemes A. The impact of personalized preventive care on health care quality, utilization, and expenditures. Popul Health Manag. 2016;19(6):389–97. https://doi.org/10.1089/pop.2015.0171.
11. Lehman AF a, Steinwachs DM. Evidence-based psychosocial treatment practices in schizophrenia: lessons from the client outcomes research team (PORT) project. J Am Acad Psychoanal Dyn Psychiatry. 2003;31(1):141–54.

12. Dieleman JL, Baral R, Birger M, Bui AL, Bulchis A, Chapin A, et al. US spending on personal health care and public health, 1996-2013. JAMA. 2016;316(24):2627–46. https://doi.org/10.1001/jama.2016.16885.
13. Stadhouders N, Koolman X, Tanke M, Maarse H, Jeurissen P. Policy options to contain healthcare costs: a review and classification. Health Policy. 2016;120(5):486–94. https://doi.org/10.1016/j.healthpol.2016.03.007.
14. Murray CJ, Atkinson C, Bhalla K, Birbeck G, Burstein R, Chou D, et al. The state of US health, 1990-2010: burden of diseases, injuries, and risk factors. JAMA. 2013;310(6):591–608. https://doi.org/10.1001/jama.2013.13805.
15. Obama B. United States health care reform: progress to date and next steps. JAMA. 2016;316(5):525–32. https://doi.org/10.1001/jama.2016.9797.
16. Seth P, Scholl L, Rudd RA. (2018). Overdose deaths involving opioids, Cocaine, and Psychostimulants - United States, 2015-2016.
17. Stuckler D, Reeves A, Loopstra R, Karanikolos M, McKee M. Austerity and health: the impact in the UK and Europe. Eur J Pub Health. 2017;27(suppl_4):18–21. https://doi.org/10.1093/eurpub/ckx167.
18. Riumallo-Herl C, Basu S, Stuckler D, Courtin E, Avendano M. Job loss, wealth and depression during the Great Recession in the USA and Europe. Int J Epidemiol. 2014;43(5):1508–17. https://doi.org/10.1093/ije/dyu048.
19. Thekiso TB, Heron EA, Masood B, Murphy M, McLoughlin DM, Kennedy N. Mauling of the "Celtic Tiger": clinical characteristics and outcome of first-episode depression secondary to the economic recession in Ireland. J Affect Disord. 2013;151(2):455–60. https://doi.org/10.1016/j.jad.2013.06.024.
20. Singla DR, Kohrt BA, Murray LK, Anand A, Chorpita BF, Patel V. Psychological treatments for the world: lessons from low- and middle-income countries. Annu Rev Clin Psychol. 2017;13:149–81. https://doi.org/10.1146/annurev-clinpsy-032816-045217.
21. Rathod S, Pinninti N, Irfan N, Gorczynski P, Rathod P. (2017). Mental health Service provision in low and middle income countries. Health Services insight 10. https://doi.org/10.1177/1178632917694350.
22. Patel V, Weobong B, Nadkarni A, Weiss HA, Anand A, Naik S, et al. The effectiveness and cost-effectiveness of lay counsellor-delivered psychological treatments for harmful and dependent drinking and moderate to severe depression in primary care in India: PREMIUM study protocol for randomized controlled trials. Trials. 2014;15:101. https://doi.org/10.1186/1745-6215-15-101.
23. Felitti VJ, Anda RF, Nordenberg D, Williamson DF, Spitz AM, Edwards V, et al. Relationship of childhood abuse and household dysfunction to many of the leading causes of death in adults. The Adverse Childhood Experiences (ACE) Study. Am J Prev Med. 1998;14(4):245–58.
24. National Institute for Care Excellence (NICE). (2019). Psychosis and schizophrenia and overview. https://pathways.nice.org.uk/pathways/psychosis-and-schizophrenia.
25. Polari A, Lavoie S, Yuen HP, Amminger P, Berger G, Chen E, et al. Clinical trajectories in the ultra-high risk for psychosis population. Schizophr Res. 2018;S0920-9964(18):30044–6. https://doi.org/10.1016/j.schres.2018.01.022.
26. Murray R. (2012). The schizophrenia commission report. http://www.schizophreniacommission.org.uk/
27. Rathod S, Kingdon D, Pinninti NR, Turkington D, Pheri P. Cultural Adaptation of CBT for Serious Mental Illness: a guide for training and practice. West Sussex: Blackwell; 2015.
28. Rathod S, Phiri P, Harris S, Underwood C, Thagadur M, Padmanabi U, Kingdon D. Cognitive behaviour therapy for psychosis can be adapted for minority ethnic groups: a randomised controlled trial. Schizophr Res. 2013;143(2-3):319–26. https://doi.org/10.1016/j.schres.2012.11.007.
29. National Access and Waiting Time Standard (AWTS) (April 2016). NHS England Publications Gateway Reference 04294 https://www.england.nhs.uk/mentalhealth/wp-content/uploads/sites/29/2016/04/eip-guidance.pdf.

30. Ising H, Kraan T, Reitdijk J, et al. Four-year follow-up of cognitive behavioral therapy in persons at ultra-high risk for developing psychosis: the Dutch early detection intervention evaluation (EDIE-NL) trial. Schizophr Bull. 2017;43(2):365–74.
31. Mohammed K, Nolan MB, Rajjo T, Shah ND, Prokop LJ, Varkey P, Murad MH. Creating a patient-centered health care delivery system: a systematic review of health care quality from the patient perspective. Am J Med Qual. 2016;31(1):12–21. https://doi.org/10.1177/1062860614545124.
32. O'Connor K, Muller Neff D, Pitman S. Burnout in mental health professionals: A systematic review and meta-analysis of prevalence and determinants. Eur Psychiatry. 2018;53:74–99. https://doi.org/10.1016/j.eurpsy.2018.06.003.
33. Johnson J, Hall LH, Berzins K, Baker J, Melling K, Thompson C. Mental healthcare staff well-being and burnout: a narrative review of trends, causes, implications, and recommendations for future interventions. Int J Ment Health Nurs. 2018;27(1):20–32. https://doi.org/10.1111/inm.12416.
34. Pradhan BK, Pinninti NR et al. (2015-2018, Unpublished data): Implementation of the Standardized Meditation Program (StaMP) for stress reduction and enhancing quality of life in health care workers.
35. Campbell H, Hotchkiss R, Bradshaw N, Porteous M. Integrated care pathways. BMJ. 1998;316(7125):133–7.
36. Rathod S, Garner C, Griffiths A, et al. Protocol for a multicentre study to assess feasibility, acceptability, effectiveness and direct costs of TRIumPH (Treatment and Recovery In PsycHosis): integrated care pathway for psychosis. BMJ Open. 2016;6:e012751.
37. Chapman SA, Blash LK, Mayer K, Spetz J. Emerging roles for peer providers in mental health and substance use disorders. Am J Prev Med. 2018;54(6s3):S267–s274. https://doi.org/10.1016/j.amepre.2018.02.019.
38. Daniels AS, Bergeson S, Myrick KJ. Defining peer roles and status among community health workers and peer support specialists in integrated systems of care. Psychiatr Serv. 2017;68(12):1296–8. https://doi.org/10.1176/appi.ps.201600378.
39. Protecting Access to Medicare Act (PAMA) 2014. https://www.acla.com/issues/protecting-access-to-medicare-act/.
40. National Council for Behavioral Health, 2019. Certified community behavioral health centers. https://www.thenationalcouncil.org/topics/certified-community-behavioral-health-clinics/
41. Kunaparaju, S., Pradhan, B.K., and Parikh S (2017): Using video-conferencing to deliver TIMBER psychotherapy for PTSD: A Case Report on an Indian Client. Poster presented in the Annual Meeting of the American Psychiatric Association, San Diego.
42. Pradhan BK, Elman I. (2017-2019, unpublished data). Combining brain stimulation (rTMS) and mindfulness therapy (TIMBER) for chronic PTSD: pilot data on 3 patients.
43. Pradhan BK and Malik S (2019). Comparative efficacy of rTMS alone and in combination with EEG-biofeedback guided mindfulness therapy (TIMBER) for resistant depression: a pilot study. Annual conference of the Philadelphia Psychiatric Society.

MIX
Papier aus verantwortungsvollen Quellen
Paper from responsible sources
FSC® C105338

If you have any concerns about our products,
you can contact us on
ProductSafety@springernature.com

In case Publisher is established outside the EU,
the EU authorized representative is:
Springer Nature Customer Service Center GmbH
Europaplatz 3, 69115 Heidelberg, Germany

Printed by Libri Plureos GmbH
in Hamburg, Germany